Springer Series on the Teaching of Nursing

Diane O. McGivern, RN, PhD, FAAN, Series Editor
New York University Division of Nursing

Advisory Board: *Ellen Baer, PhD, RN, FAAN; Carla Mariano, EdD, RN; Janet A. Rodgers, PhD, RN, FAAN; Alice Adam Young, PhD, RN*

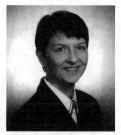

Kathleen B. Gaberson, PhD, RN, is a Professor at Duquesne University School of Nursing in Pittsburgh, PA. She has over 25 years of teaching experience in graduate, baccalaureate, diploma, staff development, and continuing nursing education programs. She has lectured, written, and consulted extensively on evaluation and teaching in nursing education.

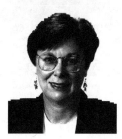

Marilyn H. Oermann, PhD, RN, FAAN, is a Professor in the College of Nursing at Wayne State University, Detroit, Michigan. She is the author of seven books and many articles on clinical teaching, clinical evaluation, and teaching strategies in nursing education. She has presented workshops, conferences, and speeches on teaching and evaluation in nursing.

Clinical Teaching Strategies in Nursing

Kathleen B. Gaberson, PhD, RN
Marilyn H. Oermann, PhD, RN, FAAN

 Springer Series on the Teaching of Nursing

Springer Publishing Company, Inc.
536 Broadway
New York, NY 10012-3955

Acquisitions Editor: Ruth Chasek
Production Editor: Helen Song
Cover design by Janet Joachim

07 06 05 04 / 10 9 8 7 6

Library of Congress Cataloging-in-Publication Data

Gaberson, Kathleen B.
    Clinical teaching strategies in nursing / Kathleen B. Gaberson and Marilyn H. Oermann.
        p.   cm — (The teaching of nursing)
    Includes bibliographical references and index.
    ISBN 0-8261-1278-1 (hardcover)
    1. Nursing—Study and teaching.   I. Oermann, Marilyn H.
II. Title.   III. Series.
    [DNLM: 1. Education, Nursing.   2. Teaching—methods.
WY 18 G112c 1999]
RT73.G26   1999
610.73'071—dc21
DNLM/DLC
for Library of Congress   99-24713
                                                                          CIP

Printed in the United States of America

This book is dedicated to our parents:
Homer and Dorothy Bollen
Laurence and Dorothy Haag

Contents

Preface

Teaching in clinical settings presents nurse educators with challenges that are different from those encountered in the classroom. In nursing education, the classroom and clinical environments are linked, because students must apply in clinical practice what they have learned in the classroom. However, clinical settings require different approaches to teaching. The clinical environment is complex and rapidly changing, and a transformed health care delivery system has produced a variety of new settings and roles in which nurses must be prepared to practice.

The purposes of this book are to examine concepts of clinical teaching and to provide a comprehensive framework for planning, guiding, and evaluating learning activities for undergraduate and graduate nursing students and health care providers in clinical settings. While the focus of the book is clinical teaching in nursing education, the content is applicable to teaching students in other health care fields. The book describes clinical teaching strategies that are effective and practical in a rapidly changing health care environment, and it examines innovative uses of nontraditional sites for clinical teaching. Although clinical evaluation strategies are addressed, for a more extensive discussion of that topic readers are referred to M. H. Oermann and K. B. Gaberson, *Evaluation and Testing in Nursing Education* (Springer, 1998).

The book is organized in three major sections. The first section of the book addresses planning for clinical teaching and contains three chapters. Chapter 1 presents a philosophy of clinical teaching that provides a framework for planning, guiding, and evaluating clinical learning activities. This philosophy forms the basis for the authors' recommendations for effective clinical teaching strategies. Chapter 2 discusses the intended and unintended results of clinical teaching; it emphasizes the need to define clear, realistic cognitive, psychomotor, and affective outcomes that guide clinical teaching and evaluation. In Chapter 3, strategies for preparing faculty, staff, and students for clinical learning are discussed. This chapter includes suggestions for selecting clinical teaching settings and for orienting faculty and students to clinical agencies.

The second section of the book explores the process of clinical teaching. Chapter 4 discusses various clinical teaching models, including traditional, preceptor, clinical teaching associate, and clinical teaching partnership models. This chapter also addresses important qualities of clinical teachers as identified in research on clinical teaching effectiveness. Chapter 5 describes the process of clinical teaching, including identifying learning objectives, assessing learning needs, planning learning activities, guiding students, and evaluating performance. Chapter 6 addresses ethical and legal issues inherent in clinical teaching, including the use of a service setting for learning activities and the effects of academic dishonesty.

The final section of the book focuses on effective clinical teaching strategies. One of the most important responsibilities of clinical teachers is the selection of appropriate learning assignments. Chapter 7 discusses a variety of clinical learning assignments in addition to the traditional patient care activity and suggests criteria for selecting appropriate assignments. Chapter 8 focuses on self-directed learning activities; it reviews various approaches to meeting the individual differences among learners through the use of multimedia and computer-assisted instruction as well as more traditional print resources. In Chapter 9, the use of learning laboratories to enhance cognitive, psychomotor, and affective learning is discussed, including suggestions for sequencing of learning laboratory and clinical learning activities.

Simulations and games are effective, creative methods of preparing students for clinical practice and at the same time add interest and variety to the learning process. Chapter 10 describes approaches to using simulations, role play, and games to teach problem solving, decision making, communication, and interpersonal skills. The ability to apply knowledge to practice, think critically about and solve clinical problems, and make sound clinical decisions are important outcomes of clinical learning. Chapter 11 discusses the use of case method, case study, and grand rounds as clinical teaching strategies to guide the development of these skills. In Chapter 12, the role of conferences and discussions in clinical learning is explored. Effective ways to plan and conduct clinical conferences, questioning to encourage exchange of ideas and higher level thinking, and the roles of the teacher and learners in discussions and conferences are presented.

Chapter 13 focuses on written assignments of various types, including short, written assignments for critical thinking, journals, concept maps, and portfolios, among others. Suggestions are made for selecting and evaluating a variety of assignments related to important clinical objectives. Chapter 14 describes effective strategies for using preceptors in clinical teaching. The selection, preparation, and evaluation of preceptors is discussed, and the advantages and disadvantages of using preceptors are explored. This chapter also discusses the use of learning contracts as a strategy for planning and implementing preceptorships. Finally, Chapter 15 suggests ways to use clinical teaching strategies effectively in diverse settings such as nurse-managed clinics, international health care settings, and home care. As the focus of health care becomes more global and population-based, settings for the delivery of care become more diverse. This chapter describes innovative ways to prepare nurses for practice in such settings.

Our thinking about and practice of clinical teaching has been shaped over many years by a number of teachers, mentors, and colleagues. It is impossible to acknowledge the specific contributions of each, but we hope that by the publication of this book, they will know how much they have influenced us as teachers. Although we now cannot identify the sources of many ideas that we have gradually formed into our own framework for clinical teaching, we wish to acknowledge the origin of two ideas discussed in this book. The concept of essential and enrichment curricula came from G. Bradley Seager, Jr. The notion that every clinical teacher has a philosophy of clinical teaching, whether or not the teacher knows it, was adapted from Elizabeth Whalen's philosophy of editing, whether or not she knows it.

Above all, we are grateful for the patience, understanding, and loving support of our husbands and children during the writing of this book: Paul Gaberson and Matthew Ammon, and David, Eric, and Ross Oermann.

Kathleen B. Gaberson
Marilyn H. Oermann

1

A Philosophy of Clinical Teaching

Every clinical teacher has a philosophy of clinical teaching, whether or not the teacher realizes it. That philosophy determines the teacher's understanding of his or her role, approaches to clinical teaching, selection of teaching and learning activities, use of evaluation processes, and relationships with learners and others in the clinical environment.

This book provides a framework for planning, guiding, and evaluating clinical learning activities of nursing students and health care providers based on the authors' philosophy of clinical teaching. That philosophy of clinical teaching will be discussed in this chapter. Readers may not agree with every element of the philosophy, but they should be able to see congruence between what the authors believe about clinical teaching and the recommendations they make to guide effective clinical teaching.

WHAT IS A PHILOSOPHY OF CLINICAL TEACHING?

A philosophy is a "belief system about human beings and their place in the world" (Csokasy, 1998, p. 101). Although it does not prescribe specific actions, philosophy gives meaning and direction to practice and provides a basis for determining whether one's behavior is consistent with one's beliefs. Without a philosophy to guide choices, a person is overly vulnerable to custom and fashion (Tanner & Tanner, 1995). Educational philosophy provides a framework for making curricular choices from among options and for understanding the implications of alternate educational decisions. The values and beliefs included in an educational philosophy provide structure and coherence for a curriculum, but statements of philosophy are meaningless if they are contradicted by actual educational practice (Dillard & Laidig, 1998; Tanner & Tanner, 1995). In nursing and other health care professions, one important type of educational philosophy is a philosophy of clinical teaching, a set of beliefs about the purposes of clinical education and the responsibilities of teachers and learners in clinical settings.

To change their practice of clinical teaching, educators first must reflect on their fundamental beliefs about the value of clinical education, the roles and relationships of teachers and learners, and how desired outcomes are best achieved. These beliefs serve as a guide to action, and they profoundly affect how clinical teachers practice, how students learn, and how learning outcomes are evaluated (Lenburg & Mitchell, 1991).

A LEXICON OF CLINICAL TEACHING

Language has power to shape thinking, and the choice and use of words can affect the way a teacher thinks about and performs the role of clinical teacher. The following terms are defined so that the authors and readers will share a common frame of reference for the essential concepts in the philosophy of clinical teaching.

Clinical

This word is an adjective, derived from the noun *clinic*. *Clinical* means involving direct observation of the patient. Like any good adjective, the word *clinical* must modify a noun. Nursing faculty often are heard to say, "My students are in clinical today" or "I am not in clinical this week." Examples of correct use include "clinical practice," "clinical instruction," and "clinical evaluation."

Clinical Instruction or Clinical Teaching

The central activity of the teacher in the clinical setting is clinical instruction or clinical teaching. The teacher does not supervise students. Supervision implies administrative functions such as overseeing, directing, and managing the work of others. Supervision is a function that is more appropriate for professional practice situations, not the learning environment.

The appropriate role of the teacher in the clinical setting is competent guidance. The teacher guides, supports, stimulates, and facilitates learning. According to Infante (1985), the teacher facilitates learning by designing appropriate activities in appropriate settings and allowing the student to experience that learning.

Clinical Experience

Learning is an active, personal process. The student is the one who experiences the learning. Teachers cannot provide the experience; they can provide only the opportunity for the experience. The teacher's role is to provide appropriate activities that will facilitate learning. However, each student will experience an activity in a different way. For example, a teacher can provide a guided observation of a surgical procedure for a group of students. Although all students may be present in the operating room at the same time and all are observing the same procedure, each student will experience something slightly different. One of the reasons teachers require students to do written assignments or to participate in clinical conferences is to allow the teacher a glimpse of what students have derived from the learning activities.

ELEMENTS OF A PHILOSOPHY OF CLINICAL TEACHING

The philosophy of clinical teaching that provides the framework for this book includes beliefs about the nature of professional practice, the importance of clinical teaching, the role of the student as a learner, the need for learning time before evaluation, the climate for learning, the essential versus enrichment curricula, the espoused curriculum versus curriculum-in-use, and the importance of quality over quantity of clinical activities. Each of these elements of the philosophy is a guide to action for clinical teachers in nursing.

CLINICAL EDUCATION SHOULD REFLECT THE NATURE OF PROFESSIONAL PRACTICE.

Nursing is a professional discipline. A professional is an individual who possesses expert knowledge in a specific domain and who uses that knowledge on behalf of society by serving specified clients. Professional disciplines are differentiated from academic disciplines by their practice component (Reilly & Oermann, 1992).

Clinical practice requires critical thinking and problem-solving abilities, specialized psychomotor and technological skills, and a professional value system. Practice in clinical settings exposes students to realities of professional practice that cannot be conveyed by a textbook or a simulation (Oermann & Gaberson, 1998). Schön (1987) represented professional practice as high, hard ground overlooking a swamp. On the high ground, practice problems can be solved by applying research-based theory and technique. The swampy lowland contains problems that are messy and confusing, that cannot easily be solved by technical skill. Nurses and nursing students must learn to solve both types of problems, but the problems that lie in the swampy lowlands tend to be those of greatest importance to society. Most professional practice situations are characterized by complexity, instability, uncertainty, uniqueness, and the presence of value conflicts. These are the problems that resist solution by the knowledge and skills of traditional expertise (Schön, 1983).

Because professional practice occurs within the context of society, it must respond to social and scientific demands and expectations. Therefore, the knowledge base and skill repertoire of a professional nurse cannot be static. Professional education must go beyond current knowledge and skills to prepare for practice in the future. Thus, clinical teaching must include skills such as identifying knowledge gaps, finding and utilizing new information, and initiating or managing change. Additionally, since health care professionals usually practice in interdisciplinary settings, nursing students must learn teamwork and collaboration skills (Oermann & Gaberson, 1998; Reilly & Oermann, 1992).

Thus, if clinical learning activities are to prepare nursing students for professional practice, they should reflect the realities of that practice. Clinical education should allow students to encounter real practice problems in the swampy lowland. Rather than focus exclusively on teacher-defined, well-structured problems for which answers are easily found in theory and research, clinical educators should expose students to ill-structured problems for which there are insufficient or conflicting data or multiple solutions (Oermann & Gaberson, 1998).

CLINICAL TEACHING IS MORE IMPORTANT THAN CLASSROOM TEACHING.

Because nursing is a professional practice discipline, what nurses and nursing students do in clinical practice is more important than what they can demonstrate in a classroom. Clinical learning activities provide real-life experiences and opportunities for transfer of knowledge to practical situations (Oermann & Gaberson, 1998). Some learners who perform well in the classroom cannot apply their knowledge successfully in the clinical area.

If clinical instruction is so important, why doesn't all nursing education take place in the clinical area? Clinical teaching is the most expensive element of any nursing curriculum. Lower student-teacher ratios in clinical settings usually make it necessary for a larger number of clinical teachers than classroom teachers. Students and teachers spend numerous hours in the clinical laboratory; those contact hours typically exceed the number of credit hours for which students pay tuition. Even if the tuition structure compensates for that intensive use of resources, clinical instruction remains an expensive enterprise. Therefore, classroom instruction is used to prepare students for their clinical activities. Students learn prerequisite knowledge in the classroom that they later apply and test in clinical practice.

THE NURSING STUDENT IN THE CLINICAL SETTING IS A LEARNER, NOT A NURSE.

In preparation for professional practice, the clinical setting is the place where the student comes in contact with the patient or consumer for the purpose of testing theories and learning skills. In nursing education, clinical learning activities historically have been confused with caring for patients. Infante (1985) observed that the typical activities of nursing students center on patient care. Learning is assumed to take place while caring. However, the central focus in clinical education should be on learning, not doing, as the student role. Thus, the role of the student in nursing education should be primarily that of learner, not nurse. For this reason, the term *nursing student* rather than "student nurse" is preferred, because in the former term the noun *student* describes the role better.

SUFFICIENT LEARNING TIME SHOULD BE PROVIDED BEFORE PERFORMANCE IS EVALUATED.

If students enter the clinical area to learn, then it follows that students need to engage in activities that promote learning and to practice the skills that they are learning before their performance is evaluated to determine a grade. Many nursing students perceive that the main role of the clinical teacher is to evaluate, and many nursing faculty members perceive that they spend more time on evaluation activities than on teaching activities. Nursing faculty seem to expect students to perform skills competently the first time they attempt them, and they often keep detailed records of students' failures and shortcomings that are later consulted when determining their grades.

However, skill acquisition is a complex process that involves making mistakes and learning how to correct and then prevent those mistakes. Because the clinical setting is a place where students can test theory as they apply it to practice, some of those tests will be more successful than others. Faculty should expect students to make mistakes and not hold perfection as the standard. Therefore, faculty should allow plentiful learning time with ample opportunity for feedback before evaluating student performance summatively.

CLINICAL TEACHING IS SUPPORTED BY A CLIMATE OF MUTUAL TRUST AND RESPECT.

Another element of this philosophy of clinical teaching is the importance of creating and maintaining a climate of mutual trust and respect that supports learning and student growth. Faculty members must respect students as learners and trust their motivation and commitment to the profession they seek to enter. Students must respect the faculty's commitment to both nursing education and society and trust that faculty members will treat them with fairness and not allow students to make mistakes that would harm patients.

The responsibilities for maintaining this climate are mutual, but teachers have the ultimate responsibility to establish these expectations in the nursing program. In most cases, students enter a nursing education program with 12 or more years of school experiences in which teachers are viewed as enemies, out to "get" students, eager to see students fail. Nursing faculty need to state clearly, early, and often that they see nursing education as a shared enterprise, that they sincerely desire student success, and that they will be partners with students in achieving success. Before expecting students to trust them, teachers need to demonstrate their respect for students; faculty must first trust students and invite students to enter into a trusting relationship with the faculty. This takes time and energy, and sometimes faculty will be disappointed when trust is betrayed. But in the long run, clinical teaching is more effective when it takes place in a climate of mutual trust and respect, so it is worth the time and effort.

CLINICAL TEACHING AND LEARNING SHOULD FOCUS ON ESSENTIAL KNOWLEDGE, SKILLS, AND ATTITUDES.

Most nurse educators believe that each nursing education program has a single curriculum. In fact, every nursing curriculum can be separated into knowledge, skills, and attitudes that are deemed to be essential to safe, competent practice and those that would be nice to have, but are not critical. In other words, there is an essential curriculum and an enrichment curriculum. No nursing education program has the luxury of unlimited time for clinical teaching. Therefore, teaching and learning time is used to maximum advantage by focusing most of the time and effort on the most common practice problems that graduates and staff members are likely to face.

Every nurse educator should be able to take a list of 10 clinical objectives and reduce it to 5 essential objectives by focusing on what is needed to produce safe, competent practitioners. To shorten the length of an orientation program for new staff, the nurse educators in a hospital staff development department would first identify the knowledge, skills, and attitudes that were most essential for new employees in that environment to learn. If the faculty of a school of nursing wanted to shorten the length of the program, they would have to decide what content to retain and what could be omitted without affecting the ability of their graduates to pass the licensure examination and practice safely. Making decisions like these is difficult, but what is often more difficult is getting a group of nurse educators to agree on the distinction between essential and enrichment content. Not surprisingly, in schools of nursing these decisions often are made according to the clinical specialty backgrounds of the faculty: the specialties that are represented by the largest number of faculty members usually are deemed to be essential content.

This is not to suggest that the curriculum should consist solely of essential content. The enrichment curriculum is used to enhance learning, individualize activities, and motivate students. Students who meet essential clinical objectives quickly can select additional learning activities from the enrichment curriculum to satisfy needs for more depth and greater variety. Learners need to spend most of their time in the essential curriculum, but all students should have opportunities to participate in the enrichment curriculum as well.

THE ESPOUSED CURRICULUM MAY NOT BE THE CURRICULUM-IN-USE.

According to Argyris and Schön (1974), human behavior is guided by theories of action that operate at two levels. The first level, espoused theory, is what individuals say that they believe and do. The other level, theory-in-use, guides what individuals actually do in spontaneous behavior with others. Individuals usually are unable to describe their theories-in-use, but when they reflect on their behavior they often discover that it is incongruent with the espoused theory of action.

Similarly, a nursing curriculum operates on two levels. The espoused curriculum is the one that is described on paper, in the self-study for accreditation or state approval and in course syllabi and clinical evaluation tools. This is the curriculum that is the subject of endless debate at faculty meetings. But the curriculum-in-use is what actually happens. A faculty group can agree to include or exclude certain learning activities, goals, or evaluation methods in the curriculum, but when clinical teachers are in their own clinical settings, often they do what seems right to them at the time. In other words, every teacher interprets the espoused curriculum differently, in view of the specific clinical setting, the individual needs of students, or the teacher's skills and preferences. In reality, faculty cannot prescribe to the last detail what teachers will teach (and when and how) and what learners will learn (and when and how) in clinical settings. Consequently, every student experiences the curriculum differently, hence the distinction between learning *activity* and learning *experience*.

QUALITY IS MORE IMPORTANT THAN QUANTITY.

Infante (1985) wrote, "The amount of time that students should spend in the clinical laboratory has been the subject of much debate among nurse educators" (p. 43). Infante proposed that when teachers schedule a certain amount of time (4 or 8 hours) for clinical learning activities, it will be insufficient for some students and unnecessarily long for others to acquire a particular skill. The length of time spent in clinical activities is no guarantee of the amount or quality of learning that results. Both the activity and the amount of time need to be individualized.

Most nursing faculty members worry far too much about how many hours students spend in the clinical setting and too little about the quality of the learning that is taking place. A 2-hour activity that results in critical skill learning is far more valuable than an 8-hour activity that merely promotes repetition of skills and habit learning. Nursing faculty often worry that there is not enough time to teach everything that should be taught, but a rapidly increasing knowledge base assures that there will never be enough time. There is no better reason to identify the critical outcomes of clinical teaching and focus most of the available teaching time on guiding student learning to achieve those outcomes.

USING A PHILOSOPHY OF CLINICAL TEACHING TO IMPROVE CLINICAL EDUCATION

In the following chapters, the philosophy of clinical teaching articulated here will be applied to discussions of the role of the clinical teacher and the process of clinical teaching. Differences in philosophy can profoundly affect how individuals enact the role of clinical teacher. Every decision about teaching strategy, setting, outcome, or role behavior is grounded in the teacher's philosophical perspective.

The core values inherent in an educator's philosophy of clinical teaching can serve as the basis for useful discussions with colleagues and testing of new teaching strategies. Reflection on one's philosophy of clinical teaching may uncover the source of incongruencies between an espoused theory of clinical teaching and the theory-in-use. When the outcomes of such reflection are shared with other clinical teachers, they provide a basis for the improvement of clinical teaching in nursing.

SUMMARY

A philosophy of clinical teaching influences one's understanding of the role of the clinical teacher and the process of teaching in clinical settings. This philosophy includes fundamental beliefs about the value of clinical education, roles and relationships of teachers and learners, and how to achieve desired outcomes. This philosophy of clinical teaching is operationalized in the remaining chapters of this book.

Terms related to clinical teaching were defined to serve as a common frame of reference. The adjective *clinical* means involving direct observation of the patient; its proper use is to modify nouns such as *laboratory, instruction, practice,* and *evaluation.* The teacher's central activity is *clinical instruction* or *clinical teaching,* rather than supervision, which implies administrative activities such as overseeing, directing, and managing the work of others. Since learning is an active, personal process, the student is the one who experiences the learning. Therefore, teachers cannot provide *clinical experience,* but they can offer opportunities and activities that will facilitate learning. Each student will experience a learning activity in a different way.

The philosophy advocated in this book contains the following beliefs. Clinical education should reflect the nature of professional practice. Practice in clinical settings exposes students to realities of professional practice that cannot be conveyed by a textbook or a simulation. Most professional practice situations are complex, unstable, and unique. Therefore, clinical learning activities should expose students to problems that cannot be solved easily with existing knowledge and technical skills.

Another element of the philosophy of clinical teaching concerns the importance of clinical teaching. Because nursing is a professional practice discipline, the clinical practice of nurses and nursing students is more important than what they can demonstrate in a classroom. Clinical education provides real-life experiences and opportunities for transfer of knowledge to practical situations.

In the clinical setting, nursing students come in contact with patients for the purpose of applying knowledge, testing theories, and learning skills. Although typical activities of nursing students center on patient care, learning does not necessarily take place during caregiving. The central activity of the student in clinical education should be learning, not doing.

Sufficient learning time should be provided before performance is evaluated. Students need to engage in learning activities and to practice skills before their performance is evaluated summatively. Skill acquisition is a complex process that involves making errors and learning how to correct and then prevent them. Teachers should allow plentiful learning time with ample opportunity for feedback before evaluating performance.

Another element of this philosophy of clinical teaching is the importance of a climate of mutual trust and respect that supports learning and student growth. Teachers and learners share the responsibility for maintaining this climate, but teachers ultimately are accountable for establishing expectations that faculty and students will be partners in achieving success.

Clinical teaching and learning should focus on essential knowledge, skills, and attitudes. Since every nursing education program has limited time for clinical teaching, this time is used to maximum advantage by focusing on the most common practice problems that learners are likely to face. Educators need to identify the knowledge, skills, and attitudes that are most essential for students to learn. Learners need to spend most of their time in this *essential curriculum*.

In clinical settings, the espoused curriculum may not be the curriculum-in-use. Although most faculty would maintain that there is one curriculum for a nursing program, in reality the espoused curriculum is interpreted somewhat differently by each clinical teacher. Consequently, every student experiences this curriculum-in-use differently. Faculty cannot prescribe every detail of what teachers will teach and what learners will learn in clinical settings. Instead, it is usually more effective to specify broader outcomes and allow teachers and learners to meet them in a variety of ways.

Finally, the distinction between quality and quantity of clinical learning is important. The quality of the learner's experience is more important than the amount of time spent in clinical activities. Both the activity and the amount of time should be individualized.

REFERENCES

Argyris, C., & Schön, D. A. (1974). *Theory in practice: Increasing professional effectiveness*. San Francisco: Jossey-Bass.

Csokasy, J. (1998). Philosophical foundations of the curriculum. In D. M. Billings & J. A. Halstead (Eds.), *Teaching in nursing: A guide for faculty* (pp. 97–115). Philadelphia: Saunders.

Dillard, N., & Laidig, J. (1998). Curriculum development: An overview. In D. M. Billings & J. A. Halstead (Eds.), *Teaching in nursing: A guide for faculty* (pp. 69–83). Philadelphia: Saunders.

Infante, M. S. (1985). *The clinical laboratory in nursing education* (2nd ed.). New York: Wiley.

Lenburg, C. B., & Mitchell, C. A. (1991). Assessment of outcomes: The design and use of real and simulation nursing performance examinations. *Nursing & Health Care, 12,* 68–74.

Oermann, M. H., & Gaberson, K. B. (1998). *Evaluation and testing in nursing education.* New York: Springer.

Reilly, D. E., & Oermann, M. H. (1992). *Clinical teaching in nursing education* (2nd ed.). New York: National League for Nursing.

Schön, D. A. (1983). *The reflective practitioner: How professionals think in action.* New York: Basic Books.

———. (1987). *Educating the reflective practitioner.* San Francisco: Jossey-Bass.

Tanner, D., & Tanner, L. (1995). *Curriculum development: Theory into practice* (3rd ed.). Englewood Cliffs, NJ: Prentice Hall.

2

Outcomes of Clinical Teaching

In order to justify the enormous expenditure of resources on clinical education in nursing, teachers must have clear, realistic expectations of the outcomes of clinical learning. What knowledge, skills, and values can be learned only in clinical practice and not in the classroom?

Nurse educators traditionally have focused on the process of clinical teaching. Many hours of discussion in faculty meetings have been devoted to how and where clinical learning took place, which clinical activities were required, and how many hours were spent in the clinical area. However, current accreditation criteria for higher education in general and nursing in particular focus on evidence that meaningful outcomes of learning have been produced. Therefore, the effectiveness of clinical teaching should be judged on the extent to which it produces desired learning outcomes.

This chapter discusses broad outcomes of nursing education programs that can be achieved through clinical teaching and learning. These outcomes must be operationally defined and stated as competencies and specific objectives in order to be useful in guiding teaching and evaluation. Competencies and specific objectives for clinical teaching are discussed in Chapter 5.

INTENDED OUTCOMES

Since the 1980s, accrediting bodies in higher education have placed greater emphasis on measuring the performance of students and graduates, holding faculty and institutions accountable for the outcomes of their educational efforts (Dillard & Laidig, 1998). Outcomes are the products of educational efforts, the characteristics, qualities, or attributes that learners display at the end of an educational program. Teachers are responsible for specifying outcomes of nursing education programs that are congruent with the current and future needs of society. Changes in health care delivery systems, demographic trends, technological advances, and developments in higher education influence the competencies needed for professional nursing practice (Boland, 1998).

The traditional approach to curriculum development as a process starts with a philosophy statement and a conceptual framework that reflects this philosophy. Program, level, and course objectives are then developed, and content, teaching strategies, and evaluation methods are selected to facilitate the attainment and assessment of the objectives. This approach to curriculum design suggests a linear, mechanistic sequence of activities, which in turn, suggests that learning takes place in the same orderly fashion. Recently, a curriculum reform movement in nursing education has focused on the need to focus on outcomes rather than process in order to improve the quality of teaching and learning. This approach suggests that an orderly curriculum design does not take into account each learner's individual needs, abilities, and learning style, and that learners can reach the same goal by means of different paths. Development of the outcome-driven curriculum begins with specifying the desired ends, then selecting content and teaching strategies that will bring about those ends (Boland, 1998).

Planning for clinical teaching should begin with identifying learning outcomes that are necessary for safe, competent nursing practice. These outcomes include knowledge, skills, and professional attitudes and values that are derived from the philosophical framework of the curriculum.

Knowledge

Clinical learning activities enable students to transfer knowledge learned in the classroom to real-life situations. In clinical practice, theory is translated into practice. In observing and participating in clinical activities, students extend the knowledge they acquired in the classroom and in self-directed learning. To use resources effectively and efficiently, clinical learning activities should focus on the development of knowledge that cannot be attained in the classroom or other settings.

As an outcome of clinical teaching, knowledge encompasses both knowing about specific facts and information and knowing how to apply theory to practice. Knowing how to practice nursing involves cognitive skill in problem solving, critical thinking, and decision making (Reilly & Oermann, 1992).

PROBLEM SOLVING

Clinical learning activities provide rich sources of realistic practice problems to be solved. Some problems are related to patients and their health needs; some arise from the clinical environment. As discussed in Chapter 1, most clinical problems tend to be complex, unique, and ambiguous. The ability to solve clinical problems is an important outcome of clinical teaching and learning. Most nurses and nursing students have some experience in problem solving, but problems of clinical practice often require new methods of reasoning and problem-solving strategies (Reilly & Oermann, 1992). Nursing students may not be functioning on a cognitive level that permits them to problem solve effectively (Klaassens, 1992). In order to achieve this important outcome, clinical activities should expose the learner to realistic clinical problems of increasing complexity.

CRITICAL THINKING

Critical thinking is an important outcome of nursing education. The recent emphasis on critical thinking skills has both affected and been affected by criteria for accreditation of nursing education programs. Many definitions of critical thinking exist, and faculty must agree on a definition that is appropriate for their program. This definition provides direction for how critical thinking is taught and how this outcome is evaluated (Nkongho, 1994; O'Sullivan, Blevins-Stephens, Smith, & Vaughn-Wrobel, 1997).

Although most educators would classify critical thinking as a knowledge outcome, some definitions of critical thinking characterize it as a composite of attitudes, knowledge, and skills (Saucier, 1995). It involves the ability to seek and analyze truth systematically and with an open mind as well as attitudinal dimensions of self-confidence, maturity, and inquisitiveness (Dexter et al., 1997). Critical thinking is a process used to determine a course of action, involving collecting appropriate data, analyzing the validity and utility of the information, evaluating multiple lines of reasoning, and coming to valid conclusions (Beeken, Dale, Enos, & Yarbrough, 1997; Saucier, 1995). Clinical learning activities help learners to develop discipline-specific critical thinking skills as they observe, participate in, and evaluate nursing care in an increasingly complex and uncertain health care environment.

DECISION MAKING

Professional nursing practice requires nurses to make decisions about patients, staff members, and the clinical environment. The decision-making process involves gathering, analyzing, weighing, and valuing information in order to choose the best course of action from among a number of alternatives. Selecting the best alternative in terms of its relative benefits and consequences is a rational decision. However, nurses rarely know all possible alternatives, benefits, and risks; thus, clinical decision making usually involves some degree of uncertainty. Decisions also are influenced by an individual's values and biases and by cultural norms, which affect the way the individual perceives and analyzes the situation. In nursing, decision making is mutual and participatory with patients and staff members, so that the decisions are more likely to be accepted (Reilly & Oermann, 1992). Clinical education should involve learners in many realistic decision-making opportunities in order to produce this outcome.

Skills

Skills are another important outcome of clinical learning. Nurses must possess adequate psychomotor, communication, and organizational skills in order to practice effectively in an increasingly complex health care environment. Skills often have cognitive and attitudinal dimensions, but the skill outcomes that must be produced by clinical teaching typically focus on the performance component.

PSYCHOMOTOR SKILLS

Psychomotor skills are integral to nursing practice, and deficiency in these skills among new graduates often leads to criticism of nursing education programs. Psychomotor skills enable nurses to perform effectively in action situations that require neuromuscular coordination. These skills are purposeful, complex, movement-oriented activities that involve an overt physical response. The term *skill* refers to the ability to carry out physical movements efficiently and effectively, with speed and accuracy. Therefore, psychomotor skill is more than the capability to perform; it includes the ability to perform proficiently, smoothly, and consistently, under varying conditions and within appropriate time limits. Psychomotor skill learning requires practice with feedback in order to refine the performance until the desired outcome is achieved (Reilly & Oermann, 1992). Thus, clinical learning activities should include plentiful opportunities for practice of psychomotor skills with knowledge of results to facilitate the skill-learning process. Psychomotor outcomes for baccalaureate students usually are expected at the level of competence in essential skills; graduate students and staff nurses generally are expected to perform at the level of proficiency or mastery of specialized skills (Infante, 1985).

INTERPERSONAL SKILLS

Interpersonal skills are used throughout the nursing process to assess client needs, to plan and implement patient care, to evaluate the outcomes of care, and to record and disseminate information. These skills include communication abilities, therapeutic use of self, and using the teaching process. Interpersonal skills involve knowledge of human behavior and social systems, but there also is a motor component largely comprising verbal behavior, such as speaking and writing, and nonverbal behavior, such as facial expression, body posture and movement, and touch. In order to encourage development of these outcomes, clinical learning activities should provide opportunities for students to form therapeutic relationships with patients; to develop collaborative relationships with health professionals; to document patient information, plans of care, care given, and evaluation results; and to teach patients, family members, and staff members, individually and in groups.

ORGANIZATIONAL SKILLS

Nurses need organization and time management skills in order to practice competently in a complex environment. In clinical practice, students learn how to set priorities, manage conflicting expectations, and sequence their work to perform efficiently (DeYoung, 1990). One organizational skill that has become an important job expectation for professional nurses in a managed care environment is delegation. Nurses need to know both the theory and skill of delegation—what to delegate, to whom, and under what circumstances (Thomas & Hume, 1998). Depending on their level (graduate or undergraduate student, staff nurse), clinical activities also provide opportunities for learners to develop leadership, followership, and management skills. These skills allow nurses to improve health care delivery through the use of power, influence, and authority (Moore, 1997).

Attitudes and Values

Clinical learning also produces important outcomes in affect—beliefs, values, attitudes, and dispositions that are essential elements of professional nursing practice. Affective outcomes represent the humanistic and ethical dimensions of nursing. Professional nurses are expected to hold and act on certain values with regard to patient care, such as respect for the individual's right to choose and the confidentiality of patient information. Additionally, they must be able to use the processes of moral reasoning, values clarification, and values inquiry. In an era of rapid knowledge and technology growth, nursing education programs also must produce graduates who are lifelong learners, committed to their own continued professional development.

Professional socialization is the process through which nurses and nursing students develop a sense of self as members of the profession, internalizing the norms and values of nursing in their own behavior. Professional socialization occurs at every level of nursing education: in initial preparation for nursing, when entering into the work setting as a new graduate, when returning to school for an advanced degree, and when changing roles within nursing (Oermann, 1997).

Students are socialized into the role of professional nurse in the clinical setting, where accountability is demanded and the consequences of choices and actions are readily apparent (DeYoung, 1990). The clinical setting provides opportunities for students to develop, practice, and test these affective outcomes. Clinical education should expose students to strong role models who demonstrate desirable attitudes and values.

Cultural Competence

Although the previous discussion attempted to classify outcomes either as knowledge, skill, or attitude, some outcomes of clinical learning are not easily categorized. One example is cultural competence, an outcome that includes elements of knowledge, skill, and attitude.

The population of the United States is becoming increasingly multicultural. If current population trends continue, by 2050 most professional nurses will work in an environment in which White European American culture no longer dominates (Zoucha, in press). Cultural competence is the ability to provide care that fits the cultural beliefs and practices of patients (Leininger, 1991). The development of this outcome begins with awareness and specific knowledge about cultural values, beliefs, rules, and traditions of the nurse's own culture as well as the patient's. Understanding and appreciating the similarities and differences between the nurse's and patients' cultures allows the nurse to be open, honest, and authentic in providing care for culturally diverse patients (Zoucha, in press). The skills of cultural competence include three major modalities that guide nursing decisions and actions: (1) cultural care preservation or maintenance actions that enable patients to maintain culturally learned lifeways in health care situations, (2) cultural care accommodation actions that help patients to adapt their specific practices in health care situations, and (3) cultural care repatterning actions that help patients to change their patterned lifeways in ways that are culturally meaningful and satisfying (Leininger, 1991; Oermann, 1997). The nurse's ability to use the "therapeutic cultural self" (Zoucha, in press) in communications and caring actions with patients is an important outcome of clinical learning. Therefore, clinical teachers should plan learning activities that will challenge learners to explore cultural differences and to develop culturally appropriate responses to patient needs.

UNINTENDED OUTCOMES

Although nurse educators usually have the intended outcomes in mind when they design clinical learning activities, those activities often produce positive or negative unintended outcomes as well. Positive unintended outcomes include career choices that students and new graduate nurses make when they have clinical experiences in various settings. Exposure to a wide variety of clinical specialties stimulates learners to evaluate their own desires and competence to practice in those areas and allows them to make realistic career choices. For example, nursing students who do not have clinical learning activities in an operating room are unlikely to choose perioperative nursing as a specialty. However, if students participate in clinical activities in the operating room, some will realize that they are well suited to practice nursing in this area, while others will decide that perioperative nursing is not for them. In either case, students will have a realistic basis for their choices.

Clinical learning activities can produce negative unintended outcomes as well. Nurse educators often worry that students will learn bad practice habits from observing other nurses in the clinical environment. Often, students are taught to perform skills, to document care, or to organize their work according to the instructor's preferences or school or agency policy. However, students may observe staff members in the clinical setting who adapt skills, documentation, and organization of work to fit the unique needs of patients or the environment. Students often imitate the behaviors they observe, including taking "shortcuts" while performing skills, omitting steps that the teacher may believe are important to produce safe, effective outcomes. The power of role models to influence students' behavior and attitudes should not be underestimated. However, the clinical teacher should be careful not to label the teacher's way as good and all other ways as bad. Instead, the teacher should encourage learners to discuss the differences in practice habits that they have observed and to evaluate them in terms of theory or principle.

Another negative unintended outcome of clinical learning may be academic dishonesty. Academic dishonesty is intentional participation in deceptive practices such as lying, cheating, or false representation regarding one's academic work. Clinical teachers often try to instill the traditional health care cultural value that good nurses do not make errors. This standard of perfection is unrealistic for nursing students and new staff members, whose mistakes are an inherent part of learning new knowledge and skills. A teacher's emphasis on perfection in clinical practice may produce the unintended result of student dishonesty in order to avoid punishment for making mistakes (Gaberson, 1997). Punishment for mistakes, in the form of low grades or negative performance evaluations, is not effective in preventing future errors (Leape, 1995). The unintended result of punishment for mistakes may be that learners conceal errors; failure to report errors can have dangerous consequences.

SUMMARY

Outcomes of clinical teaching include knowledge, skills, and attitudes that are attained through clinical teaching and learning. Current educational accreditation criteria focus on evidence that meaningful outcomes of learning have been produced. The effectiveness of clinical teaching can be judged on the extent to which it produces intended learning outcomes.
     Clinical learning activities should focus on the development of *knowledge* that cannot be acquired in the classroom or other learning settings. In clinical practice, theory is translated into practice. Knowledge outcomes include cognitive skill in problem solving, critical thinking, and decision making. *Problem-solving* ability is an important outcome of clinical teaching. Problems related to patients or the health care environment typically are unique, complex, and ambiguous, and often require new methods of reasoning and problem-solving strategies. *Critical thinking* is a process used to determine a course of action after collecting appropriate data, analyzing the validity and utility of the information, evaluating multiple lines of reasoning, and coming to valid conclusions. Critical thinking is facilitated by attitudinal dimensions of self-confidence, maturity, and inquisitiveness. Clinical learning activities help learners to develop discipline-specific critical thinking skills as they observe, participate in, and evaluate nursing care. *Decision making* involves gathering, analyzing, weighing, and valuing information in order to choose the best course of action from among a number of alternatives. Since nurses rarely know all possible alternatives, benefits, and risks, clinical decision making usually involves some degree of uncertainty. Clinical education should involve learners in realistic situations that require them to make decisions about patients, staff members, and the clinical environment in order to produce this outcome.
     Skills are another important outcome of clinical learning. Many skills have cognitive and attitudinal dimensions, but clinical teaching typically focuses on the performance component. *Psychomotor skills* are purposeful, complex, movement-oriented activities that involve an overt physical

response requiring neuromuscular coordination. They include the ability to perform proficiently, smoothly, and consistently, under varying conditions and within appropriate time limits. *Interpersonal skills* are used to assess client needs, to plan and implement patient care, to evaluate the outcomes of care, and to record and disseminate information. These skills include communication, therapeutic use of self, and using the teaching process. Interpersonal skills involve knowledge of human behavior and social systems, but there also is a motor component largely comprising verbal and nonverbal behavior. Nurses need *organizational skills* in order to set priorities, manage conflicting expectations, and sequence their work to perform efficiently. Using the skill of delegation often is an important job expectation; nurses need to know what to delegate, to whom, and under what circumstances. Clinical learning activities provide opportunities for learners to develop leadership, "followership," and management skills.

Clinical learning also produces important outcomes in *attitudes and values* that represent the humanistic and ethical dimensions of nursing. Professional nurses are expected to hold and act on certain values with regard to patient care and to use the processes of moral reasoning, values clarification, and values inquiry. These values are developed and internalized through the process of professional socialization. In an era of rapid knowledge and technology growth, nursing education programs also must produce graduates who are lifelong learners, committed to their own continued professional development.

One example of an outcome that encompasses knowledge, skills, and attitudes is cultural competence. Cultural competence is the ability to provide care that fits the cultural beliefs and practices of patients. This outcome includes understanding and appreciating the similarities and differences between the nurse's and patients' cultures that support the use of three major modalities that guide nursing decisions and actions: cultural care preservation or maintenance, cultural care accommodation, and cultural care repatterning.

Clinical learning activities also produce positive and negative unintended outcomes. Exposure to a wide variety of clinical specialties stimulates learners to evaluate their own desires and competence to practice in those areas and allows them to make realistic career choices. However, observing various role models in the clinical environment may result in students' learning bad practice habits. The unintended result of a teacher's unrealistic emphasis on perfection in clinical practice may be that learners conceal errors, with potentially dangerous consequences.

REFERENCES

Beeken, J. E., Dale, M. L., Enos, M. F., & Yarbrough, S. (1997). Teaching critical thinking skills to undergraduate nursing students. *Nurse Educator, 22*(3), 37–39.

Boland, D. L. (1998). Developing curriculum: Frameworks, outcomes, and competencies. In D. M. Billings & J. A. Halstead (Eds.), *Teaching in nursing: A guide for faculty* (pp. 135–150). Philadelphia: Saunders.

Dexter, P., Applegate, M., Backer, J., Claytor, K., Keefer, J., Norton, B., & Ross, B. (1997). A proposed framework for teaching and evaluating critical thinking in nursing. *Journal of Professional Nursing, 13,* 160–167.

DeYoung, S. (1990). *Teaching nursing.* Redwood City, CA: Addison-Wesley.

Dillard, N., & Laidig, J. (1998). Curriculum development: An overview. In D. M. Billings & J. A. Halstead (Eds.), *Teaching in nursing: A guide for faculty* (pp. 69–83). Philadelphia: Saunders.

Gaberson, K. B. (1997). Academic dishonesty among nursing students. *Nursing Forum, 32*(3), 14–20.

Infante, M. S. (1985). *The clinical laboratory in nursing education* (2nd ed.). New York: Wiley.

Klaassens, E. (1992). Strategies to enhance problem solving. *Nurse Educator, 17*(3), 28–31.

Leape, L. (1995). Reducing the incidence of adverse drug events. *Quality connection: News from the Institute for Healthcare Improvement, 4*(2), 4–7.

Leininger, M. M. (Ed.). (1991). *Cultural care diversity and universality: A theory of nursing.* New York: National League for Nursing.

Moore, K. (1997). Leadership in nursing. In M. H. Oermann (Ed.), *Professional nursing practice* (255–272). Stamford, CT: Appleton & Lange.

Nkongho, N. (1994). Critical thinking: An important outcome of nursing education. *Connections* (Spring 1994), 1.

Oermann, M. H. (1997). *Professional nursing practice* (pp. 255–272). Stamford, CT: Appleton & Lange.

O'Sullivan, P. S., Blevins-Stephens, W. L., Smith, F. M., & Vaughn-Wrobel, B. (1997). Addressing the National League for Nursing critical thinking outcome. *Nurse Educator, 22*(1), 23–29.

Reilly, D. E., & Oermann, M. H. (1992). *Clinical teaching in nursing education* (2nd ed.). New York: National League for Nursing.

Saucier, B. L. (1995). Critical thinking skills of baccalaureate nursing students. *Journal of Professional Nursing, 11,* 351–357.

Thomas, S., & Hume, G. (1998). Delegation competencies: Beginning practitioners' reflections. *Nurse Educator, 23*(1), 38–41.

Zoucha, R. (in press). Holding the keys to delivering culturally appropriate nursing care: Look within! *American Journal of Nursing.*

3

Preparing for Clinical Learning Activities

Nurse educators should consider a number of factors in preparing for clinical learning activities. Equipping students to enter the clinical setting must be balanced with preparing staff members for the presence of learners in a service setting and by respect for the needs of patients. This chapter describes the roles and responsibilities of faculty, staff members, and others involved in clinical teaching and suggests strategies for preparing students and staff members for clinical learning. Strategies for selecting clinical learning activities will be discussed in Chapter 7.

UNDERSTANDING THE CONTEXT FOR CLINICAL LEARNING ACTIVITIES

To begin preparations for clinical teaching and learning, nurse educators should reflect on the context in which these activities take place. Teachers and learners use an established health care setting for a learning environment, thus creating a temporary system within a permanent system. What are the effects of clinical teaching as a temporary system?

Over the last century, basic preparation for professional nursing has been moved from service-based training and apprenticeship into academic educational programs in institutions of higher learning. As a result of this service-education separation, the clinical teacher and students who enter a clinical setting for learning activities often are regarded as strangers or guests in the permanent social system of a health care agency (Paterson, 1997).

The clinical teacher and students in an academic nursing education program comprise a temporary system within the permanent culture of the clinical setting. Similarly, a staff development instructor and orientees may represent a temporary system. A temporary system is a set of individuals who work together on a complex task over a limited period of time. In contrast, staff members in the clinical agency have long-term membership in a permanent system with well-defined roles and identities. Although many clinical teachers view themselves as professional colleagues of nursing staff members, they are at the same time alienated from the permanent structure of the clinical agency (Paterson, 1997). Packford and Polifroni (1992) depicted the clinical teacher as straddling the gap between academia and service. In this context, clinical teachers function as diplomats and negotiators with staff members while serving as gatekeepers, buffers, and protectors of students. Often, the effect on students of these gatekeeping and protecting functions is to stifle learning. Because of faculty members' desire for credibility and acceptance by staff members, they tend to minimize students' risk-taking in an effort to prevent mistakes (Packford & Polifroni, 1992).

Consequences for clinical teachers and their students of being a temporary system in the clinical setting include territoriality, defensiveness, separateness, and inadequate communication. Both permanent and temporary systems establish territorial boundaries that are communicated through verbal and nonverbal behavior. Teachers often coach students to ask permission before using property, to appear pleasant and grateful, and to give up a patient's chart if it is requested by a physician or a staff nurse. Students often are viewed by nursing staff as the teacher's responsibility, and although students may be encouraged to use staff nurses as resources, both students and staff may avoid this contact. Teachers and nursing staff may exhibit defensiveness when their competence and professional identities are criticized by members of the other system. The separateness of the two systems may be evident in the lack of extensive interactions between them, and nursing staff and clinical teachers may fail to communicate essential information to each other. To overcome these negative consequences, clinical teachers often attempt to "court" the staff by being responsive, avoiding confrontations about patient care, and monitoring students closely to minimize errors that might aggravate staff. Some of these consequences may be avoided by a simple measure such as regular meetings between teachers and nurse managers (Paterson, 1997).

SELECTING CLINICAL SETTINGS

Clinical teachers may have sole responsibility for selecting the settings in which clinical learning activities occur, or their input may be sought by those who make these decisions. In either case, selection of clinical sites should be based on important criteria such as compatibility of school and agency philosophy, type of practice model used, availability of opportunities to meet learning objectives, geographical location, availability of role models, and physical resources (DeYoung, 1990; Stokes, 1998).

In some areas, selection of appropriate clinical settings may be difficult because of competition among several nursing programs, and nursing programs typically must contract with a variety of agencies to provide adequate learning opportunities for students. Using a large number of clinical sites increases the time and energy required for teachers to develop relationships with staff, to obtain necessary information about agencies, and to develop and maintain competence to practice in diverse settings (Reilly & Oermann, 1992).

Selection Criteria

Nurse educators should conduct a careful assessment of potential clinical sites before selecting those that will be used. Faculty who also are employed in clinical agencies may provide some of the necessary information, and teachers who have instructed students in an agency can provide ongoing input into its continued suitability as a practice site. Assessment of potential clinical agencies should address the following criteria (DeYoung, 1990; Reilly & Oermann, 1992):

- *Opportunity to achieve learning objectives.* Are sufficient opportunities available to allow learners to achieve learning objectives? For example, if planning, implementing, and evaluating preoperative teaching is an important course objective, the average preoperative patient census must be sufficient to permit learners to practice these skills. If the objectives require learners to practice direct patient care, does the agency allow this, or will learners only be permitted to observe? Will learners from other educational programs also be present in the clinical environment at the same time? If so, how much competition for the same learning opportunities is anticipated?
- *Level of the learner.* If the learners are undergraduate students at the beginning level of the curriculum, the agency must provide ample opportunity to practice basic skills. Graduate students need learning activities that will allow them to develop advanced practice skills. Does the clinical agency permit graduate students to practice independently or under the guidance of a preceptor, without an on-site instructor?
- *Degree of control by faculty.* Does the agency staff recognize the authority of the clinical teacher to plan appropriate learning activ-

ities for students, or do agency policies limit or prescribe the kinds and timing of student activities? Do agency personnel view learners as additions to the staff and expect them to provide service to patients, or do they acknowledge the role of students as learners?

- *Compatibility of philosophies.* Are the philosophies of clinical agency and educational program compatible? For example, the philosophy of a school of nursing emphasizes patients' right to self-determination, but the agency within which students are to be placed for perioperative nursing clinical practice routinely suspends patients' "do not resuscitate" advanced directives when they are scheduled for surgery. In this example, the faculty member might wish to seek another agency whose philosophy of care is more compatible with that of the school.
- *Availability of role models for students.* As discussed in Chapter 2, students often imitate the behaviors they observe in staff nurses. Are the agency staff positive role models for students and new staff nurses? If learners are graduate students who are learning advanced practice roles, are strong, positive role models available to serve as preceptors and mentors? Is staffing adequate to permit staff members to interact with students?
- *Geographical location.* Although geographical location of the clinical agency usually is not the most important selection criterion, often it is a crucial factor when a large number of clinical agencies must be used. Travel time between the campus and clinical settings for faculty and students must be considered, especially when learning activities are scheduled in both settings on the same day. Is travel to the agency via public transportation possible and safe, especially if faculty and students must travel in the evening or at night? Are public transportation schedules convenient; do they allow students and faculty to arrive at the agency in time for the scheduled start of activities, and do they permit a return trip to campus or home without excessive wait times? Does the value of available learning opportunities at the agency outweigh the disadvantages of travel time and cost?
- *Physical facilities.* Are physical facilities such as conference space, locker room or other space to store personal belongings, cafeteria or other dining facility, library and other reference materials, and parking available for use by clinical teachers and students?
- *Staff relationships with teachers and learners.* Do staff members respond positively to the presence of students? Will the staff members cooperate with teachers in selecting appropriate learning activities and participate in orientation activities for faculty and students?
- *Orientation needs.* Some clinical agencies require faculty members to attend scheduled orientation sessions before they take students into

the clinical setting. The time required for such orientation must be considered when selecting clinical agencies. If faculty members also are employed in the agency as casual or per diem staff, this orientation requirement may be waived.

- *Opportunity for interdisciplinary activities.* Are there opportunities for learners to practice as members of an interdisciplinary health care team? Will learners have contact with other health care practitioners such as physical therapists, pharmacists, nutritionists, respiratory therapists, social workers, infection control personnel, and physicians?
- *Agency requirements.* Unless the educational program and the clinical facility are parts of the same organization, a legal contract or agreement usually must be negotiated to permit students and faculty to use the agency as a clinical teaching site. Such contracts or agreements typically specify requirements such as school and individual liability insurance; competence in cardiopulmonary resuscitation; professional licensure for faculty, graduate students, and RN-to-BSN students; immunization and other health requirements; dress code; and use of name tags or identification badges. Sufficient time must be allowed before the anticipated start of clinical activities to negotiate the contract and for faculty and students to meet the requirements.
- *Agency licensure and accreditation.* Accreditation requirements for educational programs often specify that clinical learning activities take place in accredited health care organizations. If the agency must be licensed to provide certain health services, it is appropriate to verify current licensure before selecting that agency as a clinical site.
- *Costs.* In addition to travel expenses, there may be other costs associated with use of an agency for clinical learning activities. Any fees charged to schools for use of the agency or other anticipated expense to the educational program and to individual clinical teachers and students should be assessed.

PREPARATION OF FACULTY

When selection of the clinical site or sites is complete, the nurse educator must prepare for the teaching and learning activities that will take place there. Areas of preparation that must be addressed include clinical competence, familiarity with the clinical environment, and orientation to the agency.

Clinical Competence

Clinical competence has been documented as an essential characteristic of effective clinical teachers (Stokes, 1998). Clinical competence includes theoretical knowledge of and expert clinical skills and judgment in the practice area in which teaching occurs (Nehring, 1990; Oermann, 1996; Oermann & Gaberson, 1998).

Requirements for accreditation and state approval of nursing education programs often require nurse faculty members to have advanced clinical preparation in graduate nursing programs in the clinical specialty area in which they are assigned to teach. In addition, faculty members should have sufficient clinical experience in the specialty area in which they teach (Krafft, 1998). This is particularly important for faculty members who will provide direct, on-site guidance of students in the clinical area; the combination of academic preparation and professional work experience supports the teacher's credibility and confidence. Students often identify the ability to demonstrate nursing care in the clinical setting as an essential skill of an effective clinical instructor (Horst, 1988; Pugh, 1988).

Clinical teachers should maintain current clinical knowledge through participation in continuing education and practice experience. Teachers in academic settings who have a concurrent faculty practice or joint appointment in a clinical agency are able to maintain their clinical competence by this means, especially if they practice in the same specialty area and clinical agency in which they teach (Krafft, 1998; Rudy, Anderson, Dudjak, Kobert, & Miller, 1995).

Familiarity with Clinical Environment

If the clinical teacher is entering a new clinical area, he or she may ask to work with the staff for a few days prior to returning to the site with students. This enables the teacher to practice using equipment that may be unfamiliar and to become familiar with the agency environment, policies, and procedures. If this is not possible, the teacher should at least observe activities in the clinical area to discern the characteristics of the patient population; the usual schedule and pace of activities; the types of learning opportunities available to develop desired knowledge, skills, and attitudes; the diversity of health care professionals in the agency; and the presence of other learners.

Orientation to the Agency

As previously mentioned, a clinical agency may require faculty members whose students use the facility to attend an orientation program. Orientation sessions vary in length from several hours to a day or more and typically include introductions to administrators, managers, and staff development instructors; clarification of policies such as whether students may administer intravenous medications; review of documentation procedures; and safety procedures (de Tornyay & Thompson, 1987; DeYoung, 1990). Faculty members may be asked to demonstrate competent operation of equipment such as infusion pumps that their students will be using.

PREPARATION OF CLINICAL AGENCY STAFF

Preparation of the clinical agency staff usually begins with the teacher's initial contact with the agency as a basis for negotiating an agreement or contract between the educational program and the agency (Reilly & Oermann, 1992). Establishing an effective working relationship with the nursing staff is an important responsibility of the teacher. Ideally, nursing staff members would be eager to work with the faculty member to help students meet their learning goals. Indeed, in academic health centers and other teaching institutions, participation in education of learners from many health care disciplines is a normal job expectation. In reality, however, some staff members more than others enjoy working with students. Because teachers usually cannot choose which staff members will be involved with students, it is important for the teacher to communicate the following information to all staff members.

Clarification of Roles

As previously discussed, staff members often expect the instructor to take complete responsibility for the students; this expectation may extend to the instructor's being responsible for the care of patients with whom students are assigned to work. Many clinical teachers remark that if they have 10 students and each student is assigned 2 patients, the instructor is responsible for 30 individuals. These role expectations are both unrealistic and unfair to all involved parties. A "hands-off" policy has negative effects on learners, the teacher, staff members, and patients.

Although the clinical teacher is ultimately responsible for student learning, students have much to gain from close working relationships with staff members. Staff members can serve as useful role models of nursing practice in the "real world"; students can observe how staff members must adapt their practice to fit the demands of a complex, ever-changing clinical environment. At the same time, staff members often are stimulated and motivated by students' questions and the current information that they can share. The presence of students in the clinical environment often reinforces staff members' own competence and expertise, and many nurses enjoy sharing their knowledge and skill with novices. Clinical teachers therefore should encourage staff members to participate in the instruction of learners, within guidelines that teachers and staff members develop jointly. Students should be encouraged to use staff members as resources for their learning, especially when they have questions that relate to specific patients for whom the staff members are responsible.

An important point of role clarification is that the responsibility for patient care remains with staff members of the clinical agency (de Tornyay & Thompson, 1987; Infante, 1985). If a student is assigned learning activities related to a specific patient, a staff member is always assigned the overall responsibility for that patient's care. Students are accountable for their own actions, but the staff member should collaborate with the student to ensure that patient needs are met. Staff members may give reports about patient status and needs to students who are assigned to work with those patients. Students, in turn, should be encouraged to ask questions of staff members about specific patient care requirements; to share ideas about patient care; and to report changes in patient condition, problems, tasks that they will not be able to complete, and the need for assistance with tasks (de Tornyay & Thompson, 1987).

Role expectation guidelines such as these should be discussed with staff members and managers. When mutual understanding is achieved, the guidelines may be written and posted or distributed to relevant personnel and students.

Level of Learners

Staff members can have reasonable expectations of learner performance if they are informed of the students' levels of education and experience. Beginning students and novice staff members will need more guidance; staff members working with these learners should expect frequent questions and requests for assistance. More experienced learners may need less assistance with tasks but more guidance on problem solving and clinical decision making. Sharing this information with staff members allows them to plan their time accordingly and to anticipate student needs.

It is especially important for faculty members to tell agency personnel what specific tasks or activities learners are permitted and not permitted to do. This decision may be guided by school or agency policy, by the curriculum sequence, or by the specific focus of the learning activities on any given day. For example, during one scheduled clinical session an instructor may want students to practice therapeutic use of self through interviewing and active listening, without relying on physical care tasks. The instructor should share this information with the staff and ask them to avoid involving students in physical care on that day.

Learning Objectives

The overall purpose and desired outcomes of the clinical learning activities should be communicated to staff members. As demonstrated in the previous example, knowledge of the specific objectives for a clinical session permits staff members to collaborate with the teacher in facilitating learning. If students have the specific learning objective of administering intramuscular injections, for example, staff members can be asked to notify the teacher if any patient needs an injection that day so that a student can take advantage of that learning opportunity.

Knowledge of the learning objectives allows staff members to suggest appropriate learning activities even if the teacher is unable to anticipate the need. For example, an elderly patient who is confused may be admitted to the nursing unit; the staff nurse who is aware that students are focusing on nursing interventions to achieve patient safety might suggest that a student be assigned to work with this patient.

Need for Positive Role Modeling

The need for staff members to be positive role models for learners is a sensitive but important issue. As discussed in Chapter 2, teachers often worry that students will learn bad practice habits from experienced nurses who may take "shortcuts" when giving care. When discussing this issue with staff members, instructors should avoid implying that the only right way to perform skills is the teacher's way. Instead, the teacher might ask staff members to point out when they are omitting steps from procedures and to discuss with learners the rationale for those actions.

Asking staff nurses to be aware of the behaviors that they model for students and seeking their collaboration in fostering students' professional role development is an important aspect of preparing agency staff to work with learners. To accomplish this goal, instructors need to establish mutually respectful, trusting relationships with staff members and to sustain dialogue about role modeling over a period of time.

The Role of Staff Members in Evaluation

Agency staff members have important roles in evaluating learner performance. Clinical performance of learners is evaluated formatively and summatively. Formative evaluation takes the form of feedback to the student during the learning process; its purpose is to provide information to be used by the learner to improve performance. Summative evaluation occurs at the end of the learning process; its outcome is a judgment about the worth or value of the learning outcomes (Oermann & Gaberson, 1998). Summative evaluations usually result in academic grades or personnel decisions, such as promotions or merit pay increases.

Teachers should carefully explain their expectations about the desired involvement of staff members in evaluating student performance. Agency personnel have an important role in formative evaluation by communicating with teachers and learners about student performance. Because staff members often are in close contact with students during clinical activities, their observations of student performance are valuable. Staff members should be encouraged to report to the teacher any concerns that they may have about student performance (de Tornyay & Thompson, 1987; Infante, 1985), as well as observations of exemplary performance. At the same time, they should feel free to praise students or to point out any errors they may have made or suggestions for improving performance. Immediate, descriptive feedback is necessary for learners to improve their performance, and often staff members are better able than teachers to provide this information to students.

However, it is the teacher's responsibility to make summative evaluation decisions. Staff members should know that they are an important source of data on student performance and that their input is valued, but that ultimately it is the clinical teacher who certifies competence or assigns a grade.

PREPARING THE LEARNERS

Students need cognitive, psychomotor, and affective preparation for clinical learning activities. It is the instructor's responsibility to assist students with such preparation as well as to assess its adequacy before students enter the clinical area.

Cognitive Preparation

General prerequisite knowledge for clinical learning includes information about the learning objectives, the clinical agency, and the roles of teacher, student, and staff member. Additionally, faculty members usually expect students to prepare for each clinical learning session. This preparation may include one or more of the following: gathering information from patient records; interviewing the assigned patient; assessing patient needs; performing physical assessment; reviewing relevant pathophysiology, nursing, nutrition, and pharmacology textbooks; and completing written assignments such as a patient assessment or plan of care.

Teachers should ensure that the expected cognitive preparations for clinical learning do not carry more importance than the actual clinical learning activities themselves. That is, learning should be expected to occur during the clinical learning activities as well as during preclinical planning. If students receive their assignments in advance of the scheduled clinical activity, they can reasonably be expected to review relevant textbook information and to anticipate potential patient problems and needs. If circumstances permit a planning visit to the clinical agency, the student may meet and interview the patient and review the patient record. However, requiring extensive written assignments to be completed before the actual clinical activity implies that learning takes place only before the student enters the clinical area. Students cannot be expected to formulate a reasonable plan of care before assessing the patient's physical, psychosocial, and cultural needs; this assessment may begin before the actual clinical activity, but it usually comprises a major part of the student's activity in the clinical setting. Thus, preclinical planning should focus on preparations for the learning that will take place in clinical practice. For example, the teacher may require students to formulate a tentative nursing diagnosis from available patient information, to formulate a plan for collecting additional data to support or refute this diagnosis, and to plan tentative nursing interventions based on the diagnosis. A more extensive written assignment submitted after the clinical activity may require students to evaluate the appropriateness of the diagnosis and the effectiveness of the nursing interventions.

Additionally, because students often copy information from textbooks (or, sadly, from other students) to complete such requirements, written assignments submitted before the actual clinical learning activity may not show evidence of critical thinking and problem solving, let alone comprehension and retention of the information. For example, many teachers require students to complete "drug cards" for each medication prescribed for a patient. Students often copy published pharmacologic information without attempting to retain this information and to think critically about why the medication was prescribed or how a particular patient might respond to it. A better approach is to ask students to reflect on the pharmacologic actions of prescribed drugs and to be prepared to discuss relevant nursing care implications, either individually with the instructor or in a group conference.

Psychomotor Preparation

Skill learning is an important outcome of clinical teaching. However, the length and number of clinical learning sessions often are limited in nursing education or new staff orientation programs. When learning complex skills, it is more efficient for students to practice the parts first in a simulated setting such as a skills laboratory, free from the demands of the actual practice setting. In such a setting, students can investigate and discover alternate ways of performing skills, and they can make errors and learn to correct them without fear of harming patients. Thus, students should have ample skill practice time before they enter the clinical area so that they are not expected to perform a skill for the first time in a fast-paced, demanding environment (Infante, 1985). It is the responsibility of the instructor to assess that students have the desired level of skill development before entering the clinical setting.

Affective Preparation

Affective preparation of students includes strategies for managing their anxiety and for fostering confidence and positive attitudes about learning. Most students have some anxiety about clinical learning activities. Mild or moderate anxiety often serves to motivate students to learn, but excessive anxiety hinders concentration and interferes with learning (Arnold & Nieswiadomy, 1997). The role of the teacher in reducing the stress of clinical practice is discussed in more detail in Chapter 4. However, in preparation for clinical learning activities, teachers may employ strategies to identify students' fears and reduce their anxiety to a manageable level. A preclinical conference session might assess learners' specific concerns and assure students of the teacher's confidence in them, desire for their success, and availability for consultation and guidance during the clinical activities. One example of an approach to reducing anxiety prior to clinical activities in a psychiatric setting was described by Arnold and Nieswiadomy (1997). In this study, students who participated in a structured communication exercise focused on identifying and discussing their anxiety about clinical activities showed significantly lower levels of anxiety on the first day of clinical practice than students who participated in a nonstructured question-and-answer session. However, for this strategy to be effective, students must be assured that revealing their fears and doubts will not influence their teacher's evaluation of their performance (Arnold & Nieswiadomy, 1997).

Orientation to the Clinical Agency

Like clinical teachers, students also need a thorough orientation to the clinical agency in which learning activities will take place. This orientation may take place before or on the first day of clinical activities. Staff members often assist the teacher in orienting students to the agency and helping them to feel welcome and comfortable in the new environment.

Orientation should include:

- the geographical location of the agency;
- the physical setup of the specific unit where students will be placed;
- names, titles, and roles of personnel;
- location of areas such as rest rooms, dining facilities, conference room, locker rooms, public telephones, and library;
- information about transportation and parking;
- agency and unit policies;
- daily schedules and routines; and
- forms and procedures used for documentation of patient information (de Tornyay & Thompson, 1987).

In addition, students need to have a phone number where they can be contacted in case of emergency, know what procedures to follow in case of illness or other reason for absence on a clinical day, and understand the uniform or dress requirements.

Not all of this information needs to be presented on site; some creative clinical teachers have developed audiovisual media, such as videotapes or slide-tape programs, that provide a vicarious tour of the facility. If the agency uses computer software to document patient information, the instructor may be able to acquire a copy of the program and make it available in the school's computer facility. Learners can be expected to review such media before coming to the clinical site.

The First Day

The first day of clinical learning activities in a new setting is almost always perceived as stressful by students; this is especially true of learners in their initial clinical nursing course (Admi, 1997). Students' first exposure to the clinical environment either can promote their independence as learners or foster dependence on the instructor due to fear. Clinical teachers should plan specific activities for the first day that will allow learners to become familiar with and comfortable in the clinical environment and at the same time alleviate their anxiety. These activities may include tours, conferences, games, and special assignments.

Even if learners have attended an agency orientation, it is helpful to take them on a tour of the specific areas they will use for learning activities, pointing out locations such as rest rooms, drinking fountains, fire alarms and extinguishers, and elevators, stairwells, and emergency exits. The instructor should introduce learners to staff members by name and title. If students need agency-specific identification badges, parking permits, or passwords for use of the computer system, the teacher may make the necessary arrangements ahead of time or accompany students to the appropriate locations where these items can be acquired.

Special assignments may include review and discussion of patient records, practice of computer documentation, and a treasure hunt or scavenger hunt to help learners to locate typical items needed for patient care. Table 3.1 is an example of a scavenger hunt activity used in orienting students to a medical-surgical unit of a hospital. Learners may be asked to observe patient care for a specified period of time, to interview a patient or family member, or to complete a short written assignment focused on documenting an observation.

These activities may be followed by a short group conference during which students are encouraged to discuss their impressions, experiences, and feelings. The teacher should review the roles of student, teacher, and staff members and should emphasize lines of communication. For example, students need to know who to ask for help and under what circumstances, that is, when to ask questions of staff members and when to seek assistance from the teacher. Handouts summarizing these expectations and requirements are useful because students can review them later when their

Table 3.1 A Scavenger Hunt Strategy

Anywhere General Hospital
Unit 2C

Work in pairs to search for the location of the items or areas listed below. Check them off as you find them.

- Locker room
- Rest rooms
- Oxygen shut-off valves
- Fire alarms
- Fire extinguishers
- Emergency exits
- Assignment board
- Kardex™
- Patient records
- Patient teaching materials
- Nurse manager's office
- Medication carts
- Linen carts
- Kitchen
- Utility room
- Reference materials
- Conference room

---

anxiety is lower (de Tornyay & Thompson, 1987). If a dining facility is available in the clinical setting, the conference may take place in that location to allow students to relax with refreshments away from patient care areas. The conference may conclude by making plans for the next day of clinical practice, including selecting assignments and discussing how learners should prepare for their learning activities. Selection of clinical assignments is discussed in detail in Chapter 7.

SUMMARY

This chapter described the roles and responsibilities of faculty, staff members, and others involved in clinical teaching and suggested strategies for preparing students and staff members for clinical learning.

The teacher and learners comprise a temporary system within the permanent culture of the clinical setting. Consequences for clinical teachers and their students of being a temporary system in the clinical setting include territoriality, defensiveness, separateness, and inadequate communication. Clinical teachers often function as diplomats and negotiators with staff members while serving as gatekeepers, buffers, and protectors of students. The effect of these gatekeeping and protecting functions may be to stifle learning. Some of these negative consequences may be avoided by establishing and maintaining good working relationships and regular communication between instructor and staff members.

Settings for clinical learning should be selected carefully, based on important criteria such as compatibility of school and agency philosophy, type of practice model used, availability of opportunities to meet learning objectives, geographical location, availability of role models, and physical resources. Selection of appropriate clinical settings may be complicated by competition among several nursing programs for a limited number of agencies, and using multiple clinical sites increases the time and energy required for teachers to develop relationships with staff, obtain necessary information about agencies, and develop and maintain competence to practice in diverse settings. Specific criteria for assessing the suitability of potential clinical settings were discussed.

When clinical sites have been selected, educators must prepare for teaching and learning activities. Areas of preparation include clinical competence, familiarity with the clinical environment, and orientation to the agency. Clinical competence has been documented as an essential characteristic of effective clinical teachers and includes knowledge and expert skill and judgment in the clinical practice area in which teaching occurs. Teachers may maintain clinical competence through faculty practice, joint appointment in clinical agencies, and continuing nursing education activities. The teacher may become familiar with a new clinical setting by working with or observing the staff for a few days prior to returning to the site with students. In addition, a clinical agency may require faculty members to attend an orientation program that includes introductions to agency staff, clarification of policies concerning student activities, and review of skills and procedures.

Preparation of the clinical agency staff usually begins with the teacher's initial contact with the agency; establishing effective working relationships with the nursing staff yields important benefits for students. Roles of teacher, students, and staff members should be clarified so that staff members have guidelines for their participation in the instruction of learners. An important point of role clarification is that although students are accountable for their own actions, the responsibility for patient care remains with staff members of the clinical agency. Staff members also need to be aware of specific learning objectives, the level of the learner, the need for positive role modeling, and expectations concerning their role in evaluating student performance. Although staff members' feedback is valuable in formative evaluation, the teacher is always responsible for summative evaluation of learner performance.

Students need cognitive, psychomotor, and affective preparation for clinical learning activities. Cognitive preparation includes information about the learning objectives, the clinical agency, and the roles of teacher, student, and staff member. Students may be expected to prepare for each clinical learning session through reading, interviewing patients, and completing written assignments. However, requirements for extensive written assignments to be completed before the actual clinical activity may imply that learning takes place only before the student enters the clinical area.

The instructor has a responsibility to assess that students have the desired level of skill development before entering the clinical setting. When learning complex skills, it is more efficient for students to practice the parts first in a simulated setting such as a skills laboratory, free from the demands of the actual practice setting. Students should have ample skill practice time before they enter the clinical area so that they are not expected to perform a skill for the first time in a fast-paced, demanding environment.

Affective preparation of students includes strategies for managing their anxiety and for fostering confidence and positive attitudes about learning. Most students have some anxiety about clinical learning activities. Mild or moderate anxiety often serves to motivate students to learn, but excessive anxiety hinders concentration and interferes with learning. In preparation for clinical learning activities, teachers may employ strategies such as a structured preclinical conference to identify students' fears and reduce their anxiety to a manageable level.

Students also need a thorough orientation to the clinical agency in which learning activities will take place. This orientation should include information about the location and physical setup of the agency, relevant agency personnel, agency policies, daily schedules and routines, and procedures for responding to emergencies and for documenting patient information.

Students almost always perceive the first day of clinical learning activities in a new setting as stressful. Clinical teachers should plan specific activities for the first day that will allow learners to become familiar with and comfortable in the clinical environment and at the same time alleviate their anxiety. These activities include tours, conferences, games, and special assignments.

REFERENCES

Admi, H. (1997). Nursing students' stress during the initial clinical experience. *Journal of Nursing Education, 36*, 323–327.

Arnold, W. K., & Nieswiadomy, R. M. (1997). A structured communication exercise to reduce nursing students' anxiety prior to entering the psychiatric setting. *Journal of Nursing Education, 36*, 446–447.

de Tornyay, R., & Thompson, M. A. (1987). *Strategies for teaching nursing*. New York: Wiley.

DeYoung, S. (1990). *Teaching nursing*. Redwood City, CA: Addison-Wesley.

Horst, M. (1988). Students rank characteristics of the clinical teacher. *Nurse Educator, 13*(6), 3.

Infante, M. S. (1985). *The clinical laboratory in nursing education* (2nd ed.). New York: Wiley.

Krafft, S. K. (1998). Faculty practice: Why and how. *Nurse Educator, 23*(4), 45–48.

Nehring, V. (1990). Nursing clinical teacher effectiveness inventory: A replication study of characteristics of "best" and "worst" clinical teachers as perceived by nursing faculty and students. *Journal of Advanced Nursing, 15*, 934–940.

Oermann, M. H. (1996). Research on teaching in the clinical setting. In K. R. Stevens (Ed.), *Review of research in nursing education* (Vol. 7, pp. 91–126). New York: National League for Nursing.

Oermann, M. H., & Gaberson, K. B. (1998). *Evaluation and testing in nursing education*. New York: Springer.

Packford, S., & Polifroni, E. C. (1992). Role perceptions and role dilemmas of clinical nurse educators. In L. B. Welch (Ed.), *Perspectives on faculty roles in nursing education* (pp. 55–74). New York: Praeger.

Paterson, B. L. (1997). The negotiated order of clinical teaching. *Journal of Nursing Education, 36*, 197–205.

Pugh, E. J. (1988). Soliciting student input to improve clinical teaching. *Nurse Educator, 13*(5), 28–33.

Reilly, D. E., & Oermann, M. H. (1992). *Clinical teaching in nursing education* (2nd ed.) (Pub. No. 15-2471). New York: National League for Nursing.

Rudy, E. B., Anderson, N. A., Dudjak, L., Kobert, S. N., & Miller, R. A. (1995). Faculty practice: Creating a new culture. *Journal of Professional Nursing, 11,* 78–83.

Stokes, L. (1998). Teaching in clinical settings. In D. M. Billings & J. A. Halstead, (Eds.), *Teaching in nursing: A guide for faculty* (pp. 281–297). Philadelphia: Saunders.

4

Models of Clinical Teaching

In clinical practice at all levels of nursing education, students develop the knowledge needed for care of patients, a professional value system that guides their decision making in practice, and an array of technological skills. While a framework for understanding and managing health problems may be acquired in a classroom or learning laboratory, it is only in the practice setting where students begin to use these concepts and theories in caring for patients, develop clinical judgment and problem-solving skills, and test out their values with patients and families. The clinical activities in which students engage are critical for developing these competencies.

Planning the clinical activities and effectively guiding students in the practice setting require a teacher who is knowledgeable, is clinically competent, knows how to teach, relates effectively to students, and is enthusiastic about clinical teaching. The teacher also serves as a role model for students or selects clinicians who will model important professional behaviors and the role for which the student is preparing. There are different models that may be used for clinical teaching: traditional, preceptor, clinical teaching associate, and clinical teaching partnership.

QUALITIES OF EFFECTIVE CLINICAL TEACHERS

The research on clinical teaching in nursing focuses on the characteristics and qualities of the teacher important in facilitating learning in the clinical setting (Oermann, 1996). Every clinical teacher should be aware of behaviors that promote learning in the practice setting and ones that impede student learning. Findings of studies on effective clinical teaching in nursing are consistent with research in medical education and higher education in general.

Knowledge

As expected, the teacher in nursing needs to be an expert in the care of patients, families, and communities with whom students are working. This is particularly true in the traditional model of clinical teaching in which the teacher is responsible for planning and guiding student learning in practice. As new knowledge is developed from research, the teacher needs to keep current in concepts and theories about nursing, effective nursing interventions, outcomes of care to be measured and managed, new technologies and their use in nursing, and clinical knowledge derived from other fields of research applicable to the practice of nursing.

In research on clinical teaching effectiveness, students have consistently reported that the teacher must be knowledgeable about the clinical practice area and must be able to share that knowledge and expertise with them as they care for patients (Benor & Leviyof, 1997; Bergman & Gaitskill, 1990; Nehring, 1990; Pugh, 1988). There are four dimensions to this knowledge: (1) understanding concepts and theories for care of patients, (2) assisting students to *use* these concepts and theories to better understand their patients' health problems and care, (3) being up-to-date on nursing interventions and how they might be used in the care of patients with whom students are working, and (4) using this clinical knowledge to help students arrive at sound decisions about patient care.

Clinical Competence

Teachers cannot guide student learning in clinical practice without being competent themselves. Clinical competence has been reported consistently in studies as an important characteristic of effective clinical teaching (Benor & Leviyof, 1997; Bergman & Gaitskill, 1990; Cahill, 1997; Nehring, 1990; Pugh, 1988; Sieh & Bell, 1994). The best teachers demonstrate expert clinical skills and judgment. They know how to function in clinical practice and can guide students in developing clinical competencies. This quality of teaching is problematic for some faculty who teach predominantly in the classroom or change practice settings frequently. It is up to the teacher, however, to maintain clinical competence or consider a teaching model that relies more heavily on preceptors and mentors in the clinical setting rather than academic faculty.

The importance of the teacher being clinically competent and able to demonstrate nursing care in a real situation has emerged in some studies as the most important characteristic of an effective teacher, at least from the students' point of view (Benor & Leviyof, 1997; Pugh, 1988; Sieh & Bell, 1994). Associate degree (ADN) students, for instance, ranked the teacher's ability to demonstrate clinical skills and judgment as the fourth most important characteristic of an effective clinical teacher; faculty, however, did not even include it within their ranking of the 10 most important characteristics (Sieh & Bell, 1994).

Skill in Clinical Teaching

Skill in clinical teaching includes the ability of the teacher to assess learning needs, plan instruction that meets these needs within the context of the goals and outcomes of the clinical experience, guide learning so students gain essential clinical knowledge and develop requisite clinical competencies, and evaluate learning fairly. These teaching skills are described more specifically in Table 4.1.

The importance of developing clinical teaching skills cannot be underestimated. Asking appropriate questions that encourage thinking and are consistent with the students' levels of understanding, showing confidence in students, accepting their mistakes, acknowledging that each student learns at a different pace with varying amounts of guidance from the teacher, and creating an environment that is supportive of students as they develop their clinical skills enhance students' learning and development. Students need immediate and honest feedback from the teacher combined with suggestions as to how they can improve their knowledge and skills. Insufficient and only negative feedback impedes learning.

Sieh and Bell's (1994) study with 199 ADN students and 22 faculty from two community colleges emphasized the importance of these teaching skills. The most important characteristic of effective clinical teaching as reported by students was correcting their mistakes without belittling them. Not criticizing students in front of others was ranked third. Behaviors ranked high by faculty were encouraging a climate of mutual respect, giving specific suggestions for improvement, and giving constructive feedback.

Few studies have linked learning outcomes to clinical teaching practices and skills. With this goal in mind, Krichbaum (1994) explored the relationship between 24 behaviors of preceptors who were supervising baccalaureate (BSN) students in the clinical setting and achievement of learning outcomes by the students. The preceptor's use of clinical teaching behaviors was assessed by the preceptors themselves and by students. Student clinical performance was related to the preceptor's teaching skills, specifically the ability of the preceptor to adapt the instruction to the needs of the students and level of performance, structuring the clinical activities

Table 4.1 Clinical Teaching Skills

- Assesses learning needs of students, recognizing and accepting individual differences
- Plans assignments that help in transfer of learning to the clinical setting, meet learning needs, and promote acquisition of knowledge and development of competencies
- Communicates objectives and expectations clearly to students
- Considers student goals and needs in planning the clinical experiences
- Structures clinical assignments and activities in clinical practice so they build on one another
- Explains clearly concepts and theories applicable to patient care
- Demonstrates effectively clinical skills, procedures, and use of technology
- Provides opportunities for practice of clinical skills, procedures, and technology and recognizes differences among students in the amount of practice needed
- Is well prepared for clinical teaching
- Develops clinical teaching strategies that encourage students to problem solve, arrive at clinical decisions, and think critically in a clinical situation
- Asks higher level questions that assist students in thinking through complex clinical situations and cases requiring critical thinking
- Encourages students through teaching and evaluation to think independently and beyond accepted practices and to try out new interventions
- Varies clinical teaching methods to stimulate student interest and meet individual needs of students
- Guides learning and students' use of resources for learning
- Is available to students in clinical setting when they need assistance
- Serves as a role model for students
- Provides specific, timely, and useful feedback on student progress
- Shares observations of clinical performance with students
- Encourages students to evaluate their own performance
- Corrects mistakes without belittling students
- Exhibits fairness in evaluation

for students, finding opportunities to observe other nurses in practice, asking appropriate questions, and giving feedback to students.

The best clinical teachers plan assignments that reflect student needs and outcomes of the course, promote transfer of learning to the clinical setting through carefully selected teaching methods, serve as role models for students, give clear explanations, create a climate in which students are comfortable to ask questions when unsure, and demonstrate effectively procedures and clinical skills. Evaluation of performance is an important dimension of the teacher's role. Research has shown that effective teachers are fair in their evaluations of students, correct student errors without diminishing the student's self-confidence, and give prompt feedback that promotes further learning and development.

Interpersonal Relationships with Students

The ability of the clinical teacher to interact with students, both on a one-to-one basis and as a clinical group, is another important teacher behavior. In Bergman and Gaitskill's (1990) study of effective clinical teaching, interpersonal relationships with students were ranked as most important. Teachers who develop positive relationships with students

- have confidence in students;
- respect them;
- have realistic clinical expectations, considering individual differences among students;
- are honest and direct with students;
- are approachable;
- demonstrate caring behaviors; and
- provide support and encouragement.

Studies consistently suggest that the interpersonal relationship of teacher and student is critical in promoting learning in clinical practice (Krichbaum, 1994; Oermann, 1996; Oermann & Gaberson, 1998; Reeve, 1994).

Personal Characteristics of the Clinical Teacher

Personal attributes of the teacher also influence teaching effectiveness. These attributes include enthusiasm, a sense of humor, willingness to admit limitations and mistakes honestly, patience, and flexibility when working with students in the clinical setting (Oermann, 1996). Students often describe effective teachers as ones who are friendly and supportive of them. Providing an opportunity to share feelings and vent concerns about patients are other attributes of an effective clinical teacher.

Three other personal qualities important in teaching in any setting are integrity, perseverance, and courage (Glassick, Huber, & Maeroff, 1997). While these characteristics were originally used to describe the teacher as a scholar, they are just as important in carrying out the clinical teaching role. Integrity implies truthfulness with students and fairness in dealing with them in the process of learning and in clinical evaluation. The teacher develops an atmosphere of trust for students to engage in open discussions, examine alternatives, and discuss conflicting opinions with the faculty. Fairness "involves the presentation of one's own interpretations and conclusions in ways that keep open an examination of alternatives" (Glassick et al., 1997, p. 64).

In clinical teaching, faculty need to persevere in their efforts to improve on their teaching methods. They should be willing to reexamine their teaching and evaluation practices and consider better ways of designing clinical activities and guiding students in their learning. Good teachers, like good scholars, strive to perfect their teaching skills over time and avoid stagnation in their teaching approaches.

Glassick and colleagues (1997) described courage as risking disapproval, having the will to take on difficult or unpopular ideas, transcending traditional views, and imagining new questions and approaches (p. 65). These are qualities we attempt to develop in our students in clinical practice, but do we demonstrate them ourselves? Courage enables the teacher to suggest new approaches to organizing the clinical practicum, propose different methods for clinical instruction, question established clinical evaluation practices, and ask if there are better ways of teaching students and judging their clinical performance.

STRESSES OF CLINICAL PRACTICE AND RELATIONSHIP TO TEACHING

Clinical practice is inherently stressful; students face uncertainties in caring for patients and unique situations that cannot be learned in the classroom or through readings. For some students, it is stressful to provide care, particularly if they are unsure about approaches and interventions to use. Students often report that they fear making a mistake that would harm the patient. Interacting with the teacher, other health care providers, the patient, and family members also may contribute to the stress that students experience in clinical practice. Other stresses, from the students' perspective, relate to the changing nature of patient conditions, a lack of knowledge and skill to deliver care to patients, unfamiliarity in the clinical setting, working with difficult patients, and developing clinical skills (Kleehammer, Hart, & Keck, 1990; Oermann, 1998a; Oermann & Moffitt-Wolf, 1997; Reider & Riley-Giomariso, 1993; Williams, 1993; Wilson, 1994). Students in clinical courses in baccalaureate nursing programs also indicated that the paperwork required for the clinical experience was an added source of stress for them (Oermann, 1998a).

Oermann and Standfest (1997) found that stresses of students ($N = 416$) in clinical practice were not consistent across clinical courses and settings for practice. Stress was highest for students enrolled in pediatric nursing clinical courses and lowest for foundations courses. Students also may experience greater stress in clinical practice at different points in the nursing curriculum. Oermann (1998a) found, for instance, that the stress experienced by both ADN and BSN students in clinical practice increased as they progressed through the nursing program; the semester prior to graduation was the most stressful time in terms of clinical practice for both groups of students. The instructor was the predominant stress reported by students in ADN programs across all levels of the curriculum. Among BSN students the most prevalent stresses were coping with demands associated with patient care and the clinical teacher.

The finding that the teacher may be a source of added stress for students confirms the need for faculty to develop supportive and trusting relationships with students in the clinical setting and be aware of the stressful nature of this learning experience. A climate that supports the process of learning in clinical practice is dependent on a caring relationship between teacher and student rather than an adversarial one. Learning in clinical practice occurs in public under the watchful eye of the teacher, the patient, and others in the setting. By keeping the nature of clinical learning in mind when interacting with students, the teacher can begin to view the situation from the learner's perspective.

Role Modeling

Socialization is the process through which students acquire the knowledge, skills, and values for professional practice. Although there are various theoretical perspectives of professional socialization, consistent among them is the notion that through this process the person acquires necessary behaviors to function in a particular role. Socialization frequently is viewed within the perspective of role theory (Oermann, 1997a). In this process, by working with someone in the role, the student gains essential knowledge, behaviors, and values for carrying out the role.

Clinical education provides the avenue for acquiring the knowledge and behaviors for practice in a particular role, whether it is a beginning professional nurse or new role such as advanced practice nurse. This process requires learning about the role, as the initial step, and observing and working with nurses in that role, as the second step.

The clinical teacher is a role model for students (Benor & Leviyof, 1997; Wiseman, 1994), although not the only role model in this socialization process. The teacher guides the student in learning about the role and role behaviors. Many clinical teachers, however, are not practicing in the role for which students are preparing. Socialization comes from an integration of clinical and other experiences, not only from the guidance of the teacher. The experiences of students with preceptors, other nurses, and other health care providers contribute to this socialization process.

Neill and colleagues (1998) found that even beginning nursing students in clinical practice seek out mentors for answering their questions, as models for practice, and for values to emulate. These researchers suggested that clinical faculty target specific mentors for students. The mentors, who reflect the role, behaviors, and values that students are seeking to develop, can provide a model for students as they develop their own view of nursing and the role of the nurse.

MODELS OF CLINICAL TEACHING

There are different models of clinical teaching: traditional, with academic faculty directly responsible for guiding student learning in the clinical setting; preceptor; clinical teaching associate; and clinical teaching partnership. In the latter three models, preceptors, clinical teaching associates, advanced practice nurses, and others in the clinical setting provide the clinical instruction with faculty responsible for overall planning, coordinating the experience, grading clinical practice, and assuming other course-related responsibilities.

Traditional Model

In the traditional model of clinical teaching, the clinical instruction and evaluation of a group of students are carried out by an academic faculty member who is on-site during the clinical experience (Nehls, Rather, & Guyette, 1997). A benefit of this model is the opportunity to assist students in using the concepts and theories learned in class, through readings, and through other learning activities in their patient care. The teacher can select clinical activities that best meet the students' needs and are consistent with course goals and objectives. Since the clinical teacher is involved, to varying degrees, with the nursing curriculum overall, the clinical activities may be more carefully selected to reflect the concepts and theories that students are learning in the course. The faculty member, in addition, is a member of the educational system and may be more committed to implementing the philosophy of the nursing program than preceptors or faculty hired only for clinical teaching, often on a short-term basis.

Disadvantages, though, are the large number of students for whom faculty may be responsible, not being accessible to students when needed because of demands of other students in the group, the time commitment for faculty who may have other teaching responsibilities and research goals (Nordgren, Richardson, & Laurella, 1998), and teaching procedures, clinical skills, and use of technologies for which the faculty may lack expertise.

The time required for clinical teaching, in planning for the experience, supervising students in the clinical field, and evaluating their learning, should not be underestimated. Research has suggested that doctorally prepared faculty with research goals and other teaching commitments who are involved in clinical teaching have more role stress than other faculty (Oermann, 1998b). Clinical teachers experience work-related stresses that are different from faculty who teach predominantly in the classroom and learning laboratory. Oermann (1998c) examined work-related stresses of clinical teachers ($N = 226$) in ADN and BSN programs. Faculty rated the extent to which they experienced 23 potential stresses associated with clinical teaching. The predominant stresses were coping with job expectations associated with their clinical teaching roles, feeling physically and emotionally drained at the end of a clinical teaching day, job demands that interfere with activities of personal importance, heavy workload, pressure to maintain clinical competence or a clinical practice without time to do so, feeling unable to satisfy the demands of work-related constituencies (students, clinical agency personnel, patients, and others), and teaching inadequately prepared students. This study suggested that clinical teaching in the traditional model may be stressful for faculty, particularly for those involved in other types of teaching, research, and service.

Paterson (1997) described one other disadvantage of the traditional model. The teacher and students are not part of the system of care; they represent, in Paterson's words, a temporary system within the permanent culture of the clinical setting (p. 197). Faculty and students often enter the clinical setting as outsiders, yet they need detailed information about patients and their care requirements to function effectively. As such, faculty negotiate with clinical staff to ensure an effective clinical experience. Development of a climate for learning depends on this relationship between faculty and agency staff regardless of the type of setting in which students are practicing. Collaboration is a give-and-take rather than a fixed dominance of one professional over another. Working relationships between the clinical teacher and staff are essential to create an environment for learning and to take advantage of experiences available in the setting. In the traditional model of clinical teaching, faculty who are not also practicing in the clinical setting often invest extensive time in developing and maintaining these relationships.

The relationships that nursing faculty develop in the clinical setting not only are with nursing staff but also involve other health providers, particularly when the goals of the clinical education are interdisciplinary in nature. Practice in many health care systems is becoming increasingly oriented toward interdisciplinary care. Betz, Raynor, and Turman (1998) described an interdisciplinary model of clinical teaching with faculty from nursing, medicine, and allied health forming an interdisciplinary team; graduate students participate with them in planning and delivering care to clients and families. Outcomes of the clinical experience are gaining practical experience on an interdisciplinary team, learning the roles of other health professionals, and developing expanded and nursing-specific approaches to assessment and care.

Preceptor Model

In the preceptor model of clinical teaching, an expert nurse works with the student on a one-to-one basis in the clinical setting. Preceptors are staff nurses and other nurses employed by the clinical agency who in addition to their ongoing patient care responsibilities provide on-site clinical instruction for the assigned students. In addition to one-to-one teaching, the preceptor guides and supports the learner and serves as a role model (Oermann, 1997b; Stokes, 1998). A faculty member from the nursing program serves as the course coordinator, lecturer, liaison between the school of nursing and clinical setting, and resource person (Nehls et al., 1997). The faculty member, however, is typically not on site during the clinical experience. The preceptor model involves sharing clinical teaching responsibilities between faculty from the nursing program and expert clinicians from the practice setting. Guidelines for setting up a preceptorship are described in Chapter 14.

One strength of the preceptor model is the consistent one-to-one relationship of the student and preceptor, providing an opportunity for the student to work closely with a role model. This close relationship promotes socialization, bridges the gap between theory and practice, and allows students to gain an understanding of how to function in the role for which they are preparing (Kersbergen & Hrobsky, 1996). Other advantages are that students are able to work closely with a nurse who is an expert clinician, develop self-confidence, improve their decision-making skills, and learn new clinical skills under the guidance of the preceptor.

Potential disadvantages of the preceptor model are lack of integration of theory, research, and practice; lack of flexibility in reassigning students to other preceptors if needed; and time and other demands made on the preceptors. Although preceptors should be prepared educationally for this role, some preceptors may lack clinical teaching skills.

In many nursing programs the preceptor model is used exclusively at upper levels of the curriculum, often in the final clinical course, and for graduate nursing students. Nordgren and colleagues (1998) described a project that used preceptors for beginning students to address issues related to student-faculty ratios, provide individualized teaching and role modeling early in the nursing program, and allow more faculty time for scholarship. In this project beginning students were placed individually with three practicing registered nurses (RNs) at hospitals and an outpatient agency; the RNs served as preceptors and provided 36 hours of clinical instruction for the students. Evaluations of the project revealed that students developed clinical skills, expanded their knowledge base, developed their self-confidence, and gained a realistic view of clinical nursing. Using preceptors for this beginning nursing course also allowed faculty to meet their professional academic responsibilities (Nordgren et al., 1998). Considering faculty workload and scholarly activities, Packer (1994) also recommended that the preceptor model be implemented at all levels of the curriculum, not only for advanced courses and in graduate nursing programs.

Clinical Teaching Associate Model

The clinical teaching associate (CTA) model involves a staff nurse who instructs a small group of nursing students in the clinical setting collaboratively with the lead teacher from the nursing program. The CTA assumes clinical teaching responsibilities for the students. The faculty member, as lead teacher, works with the CTA to coordinate the overall clinical practicum, design the clinical experiences, assist in the evaluation of student clinical performance, and serve as a resource in undergraduate clinical teaching and mentor for the CTA (Phillips & Kaempfer, 1987; Stokes, 1998). Similar to the preceptor model, faculty may not be on site during the actual clinical activities. In return for the CTA's time, the faculty may conduct teaching for staff, may provide consultation in the clinical setting, and may assist with discharge planning or case management (Nordgren et al., 1998).

Clinical Teaching Partnership Model

The clinical teaching partnership model varies with the academic institution but is generally a collaborative relationship between a clinical agency and nursing program involving the sharing of an advanced practice nurse and academic faculty member. The advanced practice nurse teaches students in the clinical setting, often on an individualized basis, with the faculty member serving as course coordinator. The faculty member works closely with the advanced practice nurse to ensure adequate clinical activities for students. Benefits of this model are the opportunity to acquire advanced knowledge for practice, develop clinical and technological skills, and gain an understanding of the role for which the student is preparing by working closely with a person in that role. For these reasons, this is often the model of choice for graduate clinical education.

The model benefits students by pairing them with an expert in clinical practice. With this model, the advanced practice nurse collaborates more formally with academic faculty in research and scholarly activities and also may be involved in classroom teaching in his or her area of expertise. The faculty member responsible for the clinical course benefits greatly from this close interaction with an expert clinician; through this relationship the faculty member has a direct link to new interventions and technologies in practice, fosters learning by pairing the student with an expert who is in the intended role, and has more time to pursue scholarly activities.

Selecting a Clinical Teaching Model

There is no one model that meets the need of every nursing program, clinical course, or group of students. The teacher should select a model considering these factors:

- educational philosophy of the nursing program;
- philosophy of the faculty about clinical teaching;
- goals and intended outcomes of the clinical course and activities;
- level of nursing student;
- type of clinical setting;
- availability of preceptors, expert nurses, and other people in the practice setting to provide clinical instruction; and
- willingness of clinical agency personnel to participate in teaching students.

SUMMARY

Teaching in the clinical setting requires a faculty member who is knowledgeable, is clinically competent, knows how to teach, relates effectively to students, and is enthusiastic about clinical teaching. The research in nursing education over the years has substantiated that these qualities are important in clinical teaching. Students describe an effective clinical teacher as one who displays these behaviors; they describe an ineffective teacher as one who lacks these qualities.

Clinical practice is inherently stressful for students. While some clinical courses may be more stressful than others, students have identified dimensions of clinical learning that are often anxiety producing, such as fear of making a mistake that would harm the patient; interacting with the patient, the teacher, and other health care providers; the changing nature of patient conditions; a lack of knowledge and skill to deliver care to patients; and working with difficult patients. In some research, students have reported that the teacher is a source of added stress for them. These findings highlight the need for faculty to develop supportive and trusting relationships with students in the clinical setting and to be aware of the stressful nature of this learning experience. A climate that supports the process of learning in clinical practice is dependent on a caring relationship between teacher and student rather than an adversarial one. By keeping the nature of clinical learning in mind when interacting with students, the teacher can begin to view the situation from the learner's perspective.

Serving as a role model for students, or selecting clinicians who will model important professional behaviors and the role for which the student is preparing, also is important in clinical teaching. Working with a role model in clinical practice facilitates the student's own socialization into the professional role, either as a beginning nurse or when preparing for a new role such as advanced practice nurse.

The teacher also chooses a model for clinical teaching: traditional, preceptor, clinical teaching associate, or clinical teaching partnership. In the traditional model of clinical teaching, the instruction and evaluation of a group of students are carried out by an academic faculty member who is on site during the clinical experience. A benefit of this model is the opportunity to assist students in using the concepts and theories learned in class and through other learning activities in the care of patients. The teacher can select patients and plan clinical learning activities that best meet the students' needs and are consistent with course goals and objectives.

In the preceptor model of clinical teaching, an expert nurse in the clinical setting works with the student on a one-to-one basis. The preceptor, in addition to his or her ongoing patient care responsibilities, provides on-site clinical instruction for the assigned student. The preceptor also guides and supports the learner and serves as a role model. The faculty member is typically not on site during the clinical experience but has important responsibilities for the course, such as serving as course coordinator, providing the classroom instruction, serving as liaison between the school of nursing and clinical setting, and being a resource person for the preceptor.

The other two clinical teaching models described in the chapter were the clinical teaching associate (CTA) and clinical teaching partnership. The

CTA is a staff nurse who instructs a small group of students in the clinical setting collaboratively with the lead teacher from the nursing program. The clinical teaching partnership model varies with the academic institution but is generally a collaborative relationship between a clinical agency and nursing program that involves sharing of an advanced practice nurse and faculty member. The advanced practice nurse teaches students in the clinical setting, often on an individualized basis, with the faculty member serving as the course coordinator. The faculty member works closely with the advanced practice nurse to ensure adequate clinical learning opportunities for students.

There are advantages and disadvantages of each of these models. The teacher chooses a model after considering the educational philosophy of the school of nursing and faculty, goals of the clinical course, characteristics of the clinical setting, the availability and willingness of experts in the setting to provide clinical instruction, and characteristics of the students. In all of the models of clinical teaching, the teacher, regardless of whether that person is from the school of nursing or clinical setting, is critical to creating a climate for learning, supporting students as they gain new knowledge and clinical skills, and serving as a role model for them.

REFERENCES

Benor, D. E., & Leviyof, I. (1997). The development of students' perceptions of effective teaching: The ideal, best and poorest clinical teacher in nursing. *Journal of Nursing Education, 36,* 206–211.

Bergman, K., & Gaitskill, T. (1990). Faculty and student perceptions of effective clinical teachers: An extension study. *Journal of Professional Nursing, 6*(1), 33–44.

Betz, C. L., Raynor, O., & Turman, J. (1998). Use of an interdisciplinary team for clinical instruction. *Nurse Educator, 23*(1), 32–37.

Cahill, H. A., (1997). What should nurse teachers be doing? A preliminary study. *Journal of Advanced Nursing, 26,* 146–153.

Glassick, C. E., Huber, M. T., & Maeroff, G. I. (1997). *Scholarship assessed.* San Francisco: Jossey-Bass.

Kersbergen, A. L., & Hrobsky, P. E. (1996). Use of clinical maps in precepted clinical experiences. *Nurse Educator, 21*(6), 19–22.

Kleehammer, K., Hart, A. L., & Keck, J. F. (1990). Nursing students' perceptions of anxiety-producing situations in the clinical setting. *Journal of Nursing Education, 29,* 183–187.

Krichbaum, K. (1994). Clinical teaching effectiveness described in relation to learning outcomes of baccalaureate nursing students. *Journal of Nursing Education, 33,* 306–316.

Nehls, N., Rather, M., & Guyette, M. (1997). The preceptor model of clinical instruction: The lived experiences of students, preceptors, and faculty-of-record. *Journal of Nursing Education, 36,* 220–227.

Nehring, V. (1990). Nursing clinical teacher effectiveness inventory. A replication study of characteristics of "best" and "worst" clinical teachers as perceived by nursing faculty and students. *Journal of Advanced Nursing, 15,* 934–940.

Neill, K. M., McCoy, A. K., Parry, C. B., Cohran, J., Curtis, J. C., & Ransom, R. B. (1998). The clinical experience of novice students in nursing. *Nurse Educator, 23*(4), 16–21.

Nordgren, J., Richardson, S. J., & Laurella, V. B. (1998). A collaborative preceptor model for clinical teaching of beginning nursing students. *Nurse Educator, 23*(2), 27–32.

Oermann, M. H. (1996). Research on teaching in the clinical setting. In K. Stevens (Ed.), *Review of research in nursing education* (Vol. 7, pp. 91–126). New York: National League for Nursing.

————. (1997a). *Professional nursing practice.* Norwalk, CT: Appleton & Lange.

————. (1997b). Role of preceptors in clinical teaching in baccalaureate nursing programs. *Nursing Connections, 9*(4), 57–64.

————. (1998a). Differences in clinical experiences of ADN and BSN students. *Journal of Nursing Education, 37*(5), 197–201.

————. (1998b). Role strain of clinical nursing faculty. *Journal of Professional Nursing, 14,* 329–334.

————. (1998c). Work-related stresses of clinical nursing faculty. *Journal of Nursing Education, 37,* 302–304.

Oermann, M. H., & Gaberson, K. B. (1998). *Evaluation and testing in nursing education.* New York: Springer.

Oermann, M. H., & Moffitt-Wolf, A. (1997). Graduate nurses' perceptions of clinical practice. *Journal of Continuing Education in Nursing, 28,* 20–25.

Oermann, M. H., & Standfest, K. M. (1997). Differences in stress and challenge in clinical practice among ADN and BSN students in varying clinical courses. *Journal of Nursing Education, 36,* 228–233.

Packer, J. L. (1994). Education for clinical practice: An alternative approach. *Journal of Nursing Education, 33,* 411–416.

Paterson, B. L. (1997). The negotiated order of clinical teaching. *Journal of Nursing Education, 36,* 197–205.

Phillips, S. J., & Kaempfer, S. H. (1987). Clinical teaching associate model: Implementation in a community hospital setting. *Journal of Professional Nursing, 3*(3), 165–175.

Pugh, E. J. (1988). Soliciting student input to improve clinical teaching. *Nurse Educator, 13*(5), 28–33.

Reeve, M. M. (1994). Development of an instrument to measure effectiveness of clinical instructors. *Journal of Nursing Education, 33,* 15–20.

Reider, J. A., & Riley-Giomariso, O. (1993). Baccalaureate nursing students' perspectives of their clinical nursing leadership experience. *Journal of Nursing Education, 32,* 127–132.

Sieh, S., & Bell, S. (1994). Perceptions of effective clinical teachers in associate degree programs. *Journal of Nursing Education, 33,* 389–394.

Stokes, L. (1998). Teaching in the clinical setting. In D. M. Billings & J. A. Halstead, *Teaching in Nursing* (pp. 281–297). Philadelphia: Saunders.

Williams, R. P. (1993). The concerns of beginning nursing students. *Nursing &
Health Care, 14*, 178–184.
Wilson, M. E. (1994). Nursing student perspective of learning in a clinical setting.
Journal of Nursing Education, 33, 81–86.
Wiseman, R. F. (1994). Role model behaviors in the clinical setting. *Journal of
Nursing Education, 33*, 405–410.

5

Process of Clinical Teaching

Clinical teaching is a complex interaction of student and teacher within the context of the environment in which it occurs. Characteristics of the teacher and learner; the clinical environment and nature of practice within that environment; patients, families, and others for whom students are caring; agency personnel and other health care providers; and the inherent nature of clinical practice with its uncertainties all influence the teaching process. With many clinical activities, the teacher and student are outsiders to the clinical setting and are perceived as guests; this too influences clinical teaching and learning.

The process of clinical teaching is described in this chapter, but the reader should be cognizant that this process is not prescriptive. Instead, it provides a framework for the teacher to use in planning clinical activities appropriate for the learning outcomes and students, guiding students in the practice setting, and evaluating clinical performance. A framework assists faculty in creating an environment and opportunities for students to learn; the outcomes of those experiences, however, may vary considerably among students because of the many factors that influence the learning process. A framework for clinical teaching guides the teacher in decision making about clinical teaching but in no way guarantees that certain learning outcomes will occur for every student. The process of clinical teaching begins with an identification of the goals and outcomes for clinical learning and proceeds through assessing the learner, planning clinical learning activities, guiding students, and evaluating clinical learning and performance.

TEACHING AND LEARNING

Teaching is a complex process intended to facilitate learning. While the goal of teaching is to lead students in discovering knowledge for themselves, the teacher encourages this discovery through deliberate teaching actions that lead in that direction. Self-discovery does not imply a lack of structure; instead, the teacher provides structure and learning activities for self-discovery by the student.

Clinical teaching is a series of deliberate actions on the part of the teacher to guide students in their learning. It involves a sharing and mutual experience on the part of both teacher and student and is carried out in an environment of support and trust. Teaching is not telling, it is not dispensing information, and it is not merely demonstrating skills. Instead, teaching is *involving* the student as an active participant in this learning. The teacher is a resource person with information to share for the purpose of facilitating learning and acquisition of new knowledge and skills.

Learning is a process through which people change as a result of their experiences. Norton (1998) defined learning as "a process of understanding, clarifying, and applying the meanings of the knowledge acquired" (p. 212). Some people view learning as an overt and measurable change in behavior resulting from an experience; however, this view negates a change in perception and insight as learning. In the clinical setting, new insights, ideas, and perspectives may be just as critical to the student's learning and development as overt and measurable behaviors. Learning, therefore, may be a change in observable behavior or performance, or it may reflect a new perception and insight not manifested by an overt change in behavior.

The teaching-learning process is a complex interaction of these processes. The teacher is a facilitator of learning, and the student is an active participant. Serving as a facilitator does not release the teacher from teaching (Hoff, 1995). Instead, the teacher assesses learning needs, plans and organizes in collaboration with students clinical activities most likely to foster learning, serves as a resource person, and creates a supportive learning environment. The student, in turn, actively participates in learning, taking advantage of activities developed by the teacher and seeking new experiences for his or her own learning. Dunn and Hansford (1997) found that a stimulating and supportive clinical learning environment created more satisfied students.

Although teaching and learning are interrelated processes, each may occur without the other. Significant learning may result from the student's clinical experiences without any teacher involvement. Along the same line, the teacher's carefully planned activities for the students may not lead to any new learning or development of competencies. The goal of clinical teaching, though, is to create the environment and activities for learning, recognizing that each student will gain different insights and outcomes from them.

PROCESS OF CLINICAL TEACHING

The process of clinical teaching includes five steps: (1) identifying the goals and outcomes for learning, (2) assessing learning needs, (3) planning clinical learning activities, (4) guiding students, and (5) evaluating clinical learning and performance. The process is not linear, but instead each component influences others. For example, clinical evaluation provides data on further learning needs of the students, which in turn suggest new learning activities. Similarly, as the teacher works with the students, observations of performance may alter the assessment and suggest different learning activities.

Identifying Outcomes for Learning

The first step in teaching is to identify the goals and outcomes of the clinical experience. These intended learning goals and outcomes suggest areas for assessment, provide guidelines for teaching, and are the basis for evaluating learning. Often they are expressed in the form of clinical objectives or competencies and may be established for an entire course or for specific clinical activities. The objectives may specify the acquisition of knowledge, development of values, and performance of psychomotor and technological skills.

Clinical objectives often address eight areas of learning (Oermann & Gaberson, 1998); an example of an objective in each area follows. Not all clinical courses will address each of these learning outcomes, and many courses will have other types of objectives unique to the practice area.

1. Knowledge, concepts, and theories applicable to clinical practice
   Relates research on pain management to care of patients in acute pain.
2. Use of critical thinking in assessment, diagnosis, plan, interventions, evaluation of care, and other clinical situations
   Considers multiple nursing interventions, weighing the consequences of each.
3. Psychomotor and technological skills and other types of interventions
   Is competent in wound care.

4. Values related to care of patients, families, and communities and other dimensions of health care
   Respects the inherent worth and dignity of patients and families different from self.

5. Communication skills, ability to develop interpersonal relationships, and skill in collaboration with others
   Collaborates with other health providers in interdisciplinary care of children with disabilities.

6. Management of care, leadership abilities, and role behaviors
   Functions effectively as case manager for heart failure patients.

7. Accountability and responsibility of the learner
   Supports the rights of patients and families to make own decisions about treatments.

8. Self-development and continued learning
   Recognizes need for continued learning.

Some courses specify the learning outcomes in the form of competencies to be demonstrated in clinical practice rather than objectives to be achieved. Competencies are the specific abilities to be demonstrated by the learner; they often reflect the proficiencies needed to perform a particular task or carry out a defined role (Oermann & Gaberson, 1998). Typically, performance criteria are established for determining achievement of the competency. For example, performance criteria for the competency of "intravenous injection of medications" might include (1) checks physician's order, (2) confirms that medication is for intravenous (IV) use, (3) determines proper method for administering IV medication, (4) assembles equipment, (5) uses correct diluent, and (6) mixes medication in proper concentration. As can be seen with this example, competencies and their performance criteria are usually stated more specifically than are clinical objectives. Caution must be exercised in developing clinical objectives and competencies to avoid having too many considering the level and numbers of learners, clinical learning opportunities available, and time allotted for clinical practice (Oermann & Gaberson, 1998).

The objectives for clinical practice should be communicated clearly to students, in written form, and understood by them. Similarly, the teacher has an important responsibility in *discussing* these outcomes and related clinical activities with agency personnel, not *telling* them. Agency personnel need input into decisions about the clinical activities and their match with the goals, philosophy, and care delivery system of the clinical setting. With this input, the teacher may need to alter intended clinical activities and plan simulations and other types of learning opportunities for students. This is particularly true in clinical settings with no formal relationships to the academic nursing program.

Students also should have input into the clinical objectives and competencies established for clinical practice. There may be some outcomes already achieved by the students and others to be added to meet their individual learning needs and goals. The objectives for the students, therefore, need to be flexible as long as each student meets the essential clinical objectives for progression in the nursing curriculum. The same principle is true for teaching in staff development; there needs to be flexibility in the competencies established for clinical instruction as long as the nurses achieve essential skills for their practice.

Assessing Learning Needs

Teaching begins at the level of the learner. The teacher's goal, therefore, is to assess (1) the student's present level of knowledge and skill and (2) other characteristics that may influence achieving the objectives. In the first area of assessment, data are collected on whether the student possesses the prerequisite knowledge and skills for the clinical situation at hand and for completing the learning activities. For instance, if the learning activities focus on interventions for health promotion, the students first need some understanding of health and behaviors for promoting health. Changing a sterile dressing requires an understanding of the principles of asepsis. The teacher's role in the assessment of the learner is important so that students can engage in learning activities that build on their present knowledge and skills. When students lack the prerequisites, then the instruction can remedy these and more efficiently move students forward in their learning.

Not every student will enter the clinical course with the same prerequisite knowledge and skills, depending on past learning and clinical experiences. The teacher, therefore, should not expect the same entry competencies for all students. Assessment reveals the point at which the instruction should begin and does not imply poor performance for students, only that some learners may need different types of learning activities for the objectives. Assessment also may indicate that some students have already attained certain clinical objectives and can progress to new areas of learning.

The second area of assessment relates to individual characteristics of students that may influence their learning and clinical performance. Students and nurses today represent a diverse group of learners with varied cultural backgrounds and learning styles. The average age of nursing students has increased, and students bring with them a wealth of life and other experiences. In addition, many students combine their nursing education with other role responsibilities, such as family and work. Information about these characteristics, among others, gives the teacher a better understanding of the students and their responses to different learning situations. Faculty need to accept individual differences among students and use this knowledge in planning the learning activities.

Planning Clinical Learning Activities

Following assessment of learner needs and characteristics, the teacher plans and then delivers the instruction. In planning the learning activities, the main considerations are the objectives and individual learner needs. Other factors that influence decisions on clinical activities include the philosophy and goals of the nursing program, characteristics of the clinical setting, and teacher availability to guide learners.

CLINICAL OBJECTIVES

Clinical learning activities are selected to meet the objectives for clinical practice. The learning activities may include patient assignment, but care of clients is not the only learning activity in which students engage in the practice setting. The specific objectives of the experience should guide selection of learning activities. If the objectives focus on developing communication skills, then the learning activities may involve interviews with patients and families, papers analyzing those interactions, role play, and simulated patient-nurse interactions, rather than providing direct care.

LEARNER NEEDS

While the clinical objectives provide the framework for planning the learning activities, the other main consideration is the needs of the student. The activities should build on the student's present knowledge and skills and take into consideration other learner characteristics. Each student does not have to complete every learning activity; the teacher is responsible for individualizing the clinical activities so that they best meet each student's needs while promoting achievement of the objectives.

Learning activities also build on one another. Planning includes organizing the activities so they provide for the progressive development of knowledge and skills for each learner.

PHILOSOPHY AND GOALS OF PROGRAM

The philosophy of the nursing program, in terms of the faculty's beliefs about learning, teaching, and clinical practice, ultimately influences the clinical activities planned for the students. If the philosophy emphasizes self-direction and independence in learning, then opportunities should be provided in clinical practice for student choice of learning activities. The clinical learning activities should reflect values that the faculty hold about the nature of nursing practice (Mundt, 1997).

Clinical activities also should be consistent with the broad goals of the program (Fothergill-Bourbonnais & Higuchi, 1995). One of the major goals of a baccalaureate program is development of critical thinking skills. Clinical activities, therefore, need to promote critical thinking and assist students in developing clinical judgment and decision-making skills. Another program goal may be using research in practice; this goal suggests the need for learning activities in reading and analyzing research and relating the findings to patients.

CHARACTERISTICS OF CLINICAL SETTING

The size of the agency, the patient population, the educational level and preparation of nurses, their availability and interest in working with students, other types of health providers in the setting, and other characteristics of the clinical environment should be considered in planning the learning activities. Some learning activities may not be appropriate for use in certain settings. Fothergill-Bourbonnais and Higuchi (1995) emphasized the importance of faculty members working closely with agency staff in planning learning activities for students.

TEACHER AVAILABILITY

The teacher's availability to work with students in the clinical setting is one other consideration in planning the learning activities. Being available to students to guide their learning when needed is an important characteristic of an effective clinical teacher. The number and level of students in a clinical group, for instance, may influence the type of learning activities planned for a course. Beginning students and nurses new to a clinical practice area may require more time and guidance from the teacher than experienced students and nurses. Or, the teacher may be off site during the majority of the clinical experience, and the learning activities, in turn, may be more effectively planned using preceptors.

Guiding Learners in Clinical Practice

The next step in the process of clinical teaching is that of guiding learners to acquire essential knowledge, skills, and values for practice. Guiding reflects movement toward a destination where the way is unknown; it is a facilitative and supportive process that leads the student toward achievement of the outcomes. Guiding is not supervision; supervision is a process of overseeing. Effective clinical teaching requires that the teacher guide students with their learning activities, not oversee their work.

Reilly and Oermann (1992) referred to this step in the clinical teaching process as the instructional phase. With some learning activities, the teacher has a direct instructional role, for instance, demonstrating an intervention to students and questioning them to expand their understanding of a clinical situation. Other teaching activities, though, may be indirect, such as giving feedback on papers, developing a new type of postconference, and preparing preceptors for their role.

In the process of guiding learners, the teacher needs to be skilled in (1) observing clinical performance, arriving at sound judgments about that performance, and planning additional learning activities if needed and (2) questioning learners without interrogation. Observing students as they carry out their clinical activities allows the teacher to identify continued areas of learning and to determine when assistance is needed. This information, in turn, suggests new learning activities for clinical practice.

Observations of the students may be influenced by the teacher's values, attitudes, and biases. All teachers should be aware of values and biases that might affect their observations of students in clinical practice and judgments, or impressions, of that performance. Guidelines for observing students are:

- Examine own values, attitudes, and biases that may influence observations of students in clinical practice and judgments drawn about performance.
- Do not rely on first impressions, for these might change significantly with further observations of the student (Nitko, 1996).
- Make a series of observations before drawing conclusions about performance and share these with learners. Every observation is merely a sampling of the student's performance in the clinical setting; do not arrive at conclusions without observing behavior over time.
- Focus observations on the clinical objectives, competencies to be achieved, or individual goals for clinical practice set by the student. When the observations reveal other aspects of performance that need further development, share these with students and use the information as a way of providing feedback on performance.
- Discuss observations with students, obtain their perceptions of performance, and be willing to modify judgments when a different perspective is offered (Oermann & Gaberson, 1998).

The second competency essential in guiding learning activities is ability to ask thought-provoking questions without interrogation. Open-ended questions about students' thinking and the rationale they used for arriving at clinical decisions foster development of critical thinking skills, an important outcome of clinical practice. Ask questions to assess understanding of relevant concepts and theories and their use in clinical practice. Question students about different decisions possible in a clinical situation, consequences of each decision, the decision they would make, and their rationale; about different problems and solutions possible; and about assumptions underlying their thinking. Ask them to describe other possible views of the clinical situation and other interventions that might be possible (Oermann, 1997, 1998a). Questions should encourage the learner to think beyond the obvious. What else is possible in this situation? What alternate perspectives might be offered?

The way in which questions are asked, however, is significant. The purpose of questions is to give feedback to students and to promote critical thinking, not to drill them. In the beginning of a clinical course, discuss the purpose of questioning and its importance in developing their critical thinking ability. Demonstrate the type of questions to be asked and answers possible. Since questioning is for instructional purposes, students need to be comfortable that their responses will not influence their clinical grades. Instead, the questions asked and answers given are an essential part of the teaching process, to promote learning and development of critical thinking skills, not for grading purposes. Only with this framework will students be comfortable in responding to questions and evaluating alternate perspectives using the teacher as a resource.

Evaluating Clinical Learning and Performance

The remaining component of the clinical teaching process is evaluation. Clinical evaluation serves two purposes: formative and summative. Through formative evaluation the teacher monitors student progress toward meeting the clinical objectives and demonstrating competency in clinical practice. Formative evaluation provides information about further learning needs of students and where additional clinical instruction is needed. Clinical evaluation that is formative is not intended for grading purposes; instead, it is designed to diagnose learning needs as a basis for further instruction.

Summative evaluation, in contrast, takes place at the end of the learning process to ascertain if the objectives have been achieved and competencies developed (Oermann & Gaberson, 1998). Summative evaluation provides the basis for determining grades in clinical practice or certifying competency. It occurs at the completion of a course, an educational program, orientation, and other types of programs. This type of clinical evaluation determines what *has been* learned rather than what *can be* learned.

In deciding on methods to use for clinical evaluation, Oermann and Gaberson (1998) identified five factors to consider:

1. The evaluation methods should determine how well students are meeting the clinical objectives or competencies, if the purpose is formative, or the extent to which they achieved these objectives, if the purpose is summative. In deciding on the evaluation methods, think first about the clinical objectives to be evaluated, then ask which method or methods would provide data on them. The process involves matching the evaluation strategies to the clinical objectives or competencies.
2. Typically there are different evaluation methods that could be used for any given objectives or competencies. The teacher should not rely on one method only, such as a rating scale, and instead should choose the most appropriate methods for the objectives and students. Varying the evaluation strategies also provides a broader data base for judging student performance.
3. The evaluation methods should be appropriate for the type of clinical activities in which students engage. For example, a rating scale is intended for rating behaviors that are observed by the teacher or some other expert. If the clinical activities are such that the teacher has limited opportunity to observe the behaviors to be rated, then this method is inappropriate. Other evaluation methods, such as written assignments, may be more effective.
4. It is important to be clear about whether the evaluation is for formative purposes or summative evaluation and to communicate this to students. If the intent is formative evaluation, then the methods provide feedback for further learning and are not included in the clinical grade.
5. In addition to the appropriateness of the method for the clinical activities, also consider faculty time for completing the evaluation, providing feedback, and determining a grade, if intended for summative evaluation (Oermann & Gaberson, 1998). The evaluation methods should not burden either the teacher or the student.

CLINICAL EVALUATION METHODS

There are many clinical evaluation methods from which to choose. These methods include:

Rating Scale. A rating scale provides a means of recording the teacher's observations and judgments about the performance of the students in clinical practice. It typically includes clinical objectives, behaviors, or competencies to be demonstrated in clinical practice and a scale for rating the performance of them (Oermann & Gaberson, 1998). The teacher observes the performance, then rates it on a scale. Scales may be multidimensional such as A, B, C, D, E, or outstanding, very good, good, fair, poor; two-dimensional, such as pass-fail or satisfactory-unsatisfactory; and other types. Bondy's Criterion Matrix allows the teacher to describe and rate the learner's performance on an outcome based on its appropriateness, qualitative aspects of the performance, and the assistance needed, using a 5-point scale (Bondy, Jenkins, Seymour, Lancaster, & Ishee, 1997; Krichbaum, Rowan, Duckett, Ryden, & Savik, 1994). The format of a rating scale is shown in Table 5.1.

While rating scales are widely used, they are not without problems. Sometimes the clinical learning activities are not designed for observation and rating of performance. Rating scales are only effective if the

Table 5.1 Format of Pass-Fail Rating Scale

Nursing Care of Children Clinical Performance Evaluation		
Name_____ Date_____		
OBJECTIVE	P	F
1. Delivers care to children with varying health problems and needs		
A. Assesses individual needs of the child considering developmental level	—	—
B. Plans care to meet the needs of the child and family	—	—
C. Uses interventions based on research and scientific rationale	—	—
D. Evaluates the effectiveness of nursing care	—	—
E. Includes the family in planning and implementing care for the child	—	—
2. Participates in health teaching for children and their families		
A. Identifies learning needs of the child and family members	—	—
B. Teaches the child and family about care for present health problems and for health promotion	—	—

Note: P = Pass, F = Fail

teacher, or another expert, has an opportunity to observe performance over a period of time. Frequently, the learning activities are not designed in this way, and as a result other evaluation methods may be more appropriate.

Observing behavior and rating its quality are a subjective process, and teachers and students may vary widely in their judgments. A clinical objective that specifies "Collects comprehensive data from patients and families" is influenced by the teacher's and the individual student's judgments of comprehensiveness. Other values and biases of the teacher may affect the data collected and resulting judgments of clinical performance.

One other problem in using rating scales is that each observation is only a sampling of the student's performance. The teacher might observe the student at a later point and develop a different impression of the student's competencies. Rating scales are often more effective if combined with other evaluation strategies that do not rely on observation of performance.

Checklist. A checklist includes a list of steps to be followed in performing a procedure or carrying out a specific technique or intervention. The behaviors to be observed are more specific than a rating scale, and generally the teacher checks whether or not they were present during performance (Nitko, 1996). The checklist should not include every possible step in a procedure, but instead should focus on critical steps and their sequence (see Table 5.2).

Anecdotal note. An anecdotal note is a narrative description of the teacher's observations of students in clinical practice. The anecdotal note may describe only the behaviors observed, or it also may include the teacher's interpretations or judgments about the performance. Gronlund (1993) recommended keeping the description of the observed behavior separate from the interpretation. The information recorded in the anecdotal note should reflect meaningful incidents, should be recorded as soon as possible after the observation was made, and should contain enough information to be understood at a later time (Gronlund, 1993).

Observations made of students and recorded in anecdotal notes should always be discussed with students, allowing for student input into the observations made and teacher's interpretation of them. Anecdotal notes are valuable for giving feedback to learners and gathering their own perceptions of performance.

Simulation. Simulations provide experiences for students without the constraints of a real-life situation. With a simulation students can think through clinical scenarios and provide care to a hypothetical patient prior *med-adm steps!* (handwritten annotation)

Table 5.2 Sample Checklist

Student Name _____

Instructions to teacher/examiner: Observe the student performing the following procedure and check the steps completed properly by the student. Check only those steps that the student performed properly. After competing the checklist, discuss performance with the student, reviewing aspects of the procedure to be improved.

IV Injection of Medication

☐ Checks physician's order.

☐ Checks that medication is for IV use and states this if asked by teacher/examiner.

☐ States proper method for administering the IV medication.

☐ Assembles appropriate equipment.

☐ Uses correct diluent.

☐ Mixes IV medication in proper concentration.

☐ Cleans site properly.

☐ Administers medication at correct rate.

☐ Flushes tubing.

☐ Documents IV medication correctly on flow sheet.

From Oermann, M. H., & Gaberson, K. (1998). *Evaluation and testing in nursing education*, p. 184. Copyright (c) 1998 by Springer Publishing Company. Reprinted with permission.

to experience in the actual situation. Another advantage in terms of clinical evaluation is that simulations enable the teacher to assess specific competencies without waiting for learning opportunities to arise in the clinical setting (Gomez, Lobodzinski, & West, 1998). While simulations may be graded, they are most effective for formative evaluation. Simulations may be in paper-and-pencil format; use multimedia, such as videotapes and interactive video; involve computer simulations; and use models. Developing simulations for clinical teaching is described more fully in Chapter 10.

Role play. Designed for formative evaluation only, role play enables a learner to portray a role and assess his or her performance in that role. Role play is most appropriate for clinical objectives on developing communication skills, interpersonal relationships, and working with other health providers (Reilly & Oermann, 1992).

Media Clip. Short segments of multimedia for students to critique, answer questions about, or respond to in some way provide another means of evaluating clinical learning outcomes. Media clips should be short, and students should be aware of the objectives in advance so they can focus their observations. Media clips showing clinical scenarios are particularly valuable for evaluating critical thinking and problem-solving skills. Students may be asked to analyze the scenario using relevant concepts and theories, identify all possible problems, propose additional data they would collect, suggest multiple interventions, and consider the various decisions possible and the consequences of each.

Problem-solving strategies. There are three types of problem-solving strategies appropriate for clinical evaluation: (1) short descriptions of clinical situations for students to identify problems and solutions, (2) decision-making scenarios requiring one or more decisions as part of the analysis, and (3) critical incidents in which students analyze a critical event and identify actions to take (Oermann & Gaberson, 1998). These strategies may be completed in small groups or individually. Examples of each type are shown in Table 5.3.

Case study. A case study is a hypothetical or real-life situation that students analyze and prepare responses to, usually in written form. Case studies are typically longer descriptions of patient situations than would be found with problem-solving strategies and are more comprehensive.

Written assignment. Written assignments accompanying the clinical learning activities are effective strategies for evaluating students' learning in clinical practice. Depending on the type of assignment, they may be geared to evaluating students' ability to apply concepts and theories to clinical situations; their problem-solving, decision-making, and critical thinking skills; and their writing skill. There are many types of written assignments appropriate for clinical evaluation; these are discussed in Chapter 13.

Journal. Journals provide an opportunity for students to describe their clinical experiences and document their responses to clinical learning activities. Brown and Sorrell (1993) recommended journals to enable students to "think aloud" and record their perceptions of clinical experiences. Journals are not intended for evaluating writing skills, but they provide an opportunity for learners to describe their feelings (Callister, 1993), react to clinical experiences, gain ability to critique positions and issues (Hodges, 1996), communicate with the teacher, and document their learning and development of critical thinking skills in clinical practice (Sedlak, 1992, 1997). Journals are best used to provide feedback to students, not for grading clinical performance.

Table 5.3 Problem-Solving Strategies

Situation
Mr. S is admitted with worsening COPD. On admission Mr. S tells
the nurse that he is more short of breath than usual, he is constantly
coughing large amounts of thick green phlegm, and his chest hurts
from coughing. On physical examination the nurse finds diminished
breath sounds.

  1. What problems do you anticipate for Mr. S? List all possible problems.
  2. What additional data would you collect from Mr. S? Why is this information important to establish the nursing diagnoses and for your care planning?
  3. Describe three nursing interventions for Mr. S. Provide a rationale for each.

Decision Making
You are completing your first home visit with Mrs. P, a 92-year-old
with multiple health problems. She tells you, "Living alone like this
is not worth it. My daughter never visits me. I'd be better off dead."

  1. List three possible responses you could make to Mrs. P.
  2. Which response would you choose? Why?
  3. When you return to the agency, you need to decide how to handle this situation. Describe two different approaches you could take and the consequences of each. What would you do? Why?

Critical Incident
Your patient is becoming more confused and pulls out her chest tube.

  1. What would you do first? Why?

Portfolio. A portfolio is a collection of projects that students complete in
clinical practice that document their learning and development of knowledge and skills. Students typically engage in these projects over a significant period of time (Bott, 1996). Since the products in the portfolio provide
documentation of student learning in clinical practice, portfolios are valuable for clinical evaluation.

There are two types of portfolios: (1) best-work and (2) growth and learning (Nitko, 1996). Best-work portfolios include projects that reflect the "best work" of the student in clinical practice. In these portfolios projects demonstrate that the student has met specific clinical objectives and competencies and has achieved at a high level in clinical practice. Best-work portfolios are appropriate for summative clinical evaluation (Oermann & Gaberson, 1998). Growth and learning portfolios are intended for monitoring students' progress in clinical practice; they also allow students to evaluate their own progress in meeting the clinical objectives.

Clinical conference. Conferences with students are another means of evaluating clinical learning outcomes. Conferences may be one-to-one discussions with learners or in a small group format. Quinn (1995) identified five outcomes of small group discussion and work: (1) intellectual—trying out new ideas, analyzing issues, and relating theory to practice; (2) affective—encouraging self-evaluation and personal development; (3) social—developing sensitivity to others; (4) expressive—developing communication skills and ability to debate; and (5) experiential—providing an opportunity to reflect on experiences.

The type of conference to be evaluated depends on the clinical objectives. Some conferences might be clinically focused and involve discussions about clients' care and other aspects of practice; these clinical conferences may be nursing or interdisciplinary in focus. Reilly and Oermann (1992) described issue conferences as discussions on clinical practice, professional, cultural, social, economic, and political issues. Conferences also may be used to assess critical thinking abilities and skill in analyzing significant incidents in practice in a group format (Brookfield, 1995).

Clinical examination. Clinical examinations are structured evaluations of clinical performance conducted in a laboratory setting, thereby providing for greater control over the environment and limiting distractions (Oermann & Gaberson, 1998). Clinical examinations are designed for evaluating clinical performance at the end of a course, orientation, and other programs as a summative evaluation method. Clinical exams often include several evaluation methods, such as viewing media, demonstrating procedures, and completing written assignments and tests. The procedures and techniques carried out in the laboratory are evaluated by the teacher or an examiner and may be videotaped for later ratings. Borbasi and Koop (1994) described the Objective Structured Clinical Examination as a simulated environment with "pretend" patients to represent actual clinical conditions. Students progress through stations, where they perform specific clinical skills evaluated by the teacher using checklists.

Self-evaluation. Skill in self-evaluation develops over time as learners gain clinical knowledge and experience. While self-evaluation begins with the first clinical course, students typically need much guidance in assessing their own performance; in beginning practice, they are unsure of the behaviors and competencies to be developed. Guidelines for helping students develop skill in self-evaluation include:

- Discuss the students' clinical performance with them and explain how this evaluation relates explicitly to the clinical objectives and competencies.
- Ask students to describe their perceptions of performance in relation to the same objectives and competencies.
- Discuss any discrepancies in assessment of clinical performance and propose reasons why perceptions may be different.
- Identify strengths and areas for future learning from both the teacher's and the student's perspectives.
- Develop with students additional learning activities that would be valuable for improving performance.

Developing skill in self-evaluation is critical for nurses to remain competent in practice as the demands of that practice change and take advantage of new roles and opportunities in nursing. Regardless of the practice setting, nurses need the ability to evaluate their own knowledge and skills for practice, to know about resources available for development of new competencies for practice, and to be willing to engage in this self-assessment (Oermann, 1998b). Self-evaluation among students and nurses alike is appropriate only for formative evaluation.

SUMMARY

The process of clinical teaching begins with an identification of the goals and outcomes for clinical learning and proceeds through assessing the learner, planning clinical learning activities, guiding students, and evaluating clinical learning and performance. The goals and outcomes suggest areas for assessment, provide guidelines for teaching, and are the basis for evaluating learning. Often they are expressed in the form of clinical objectives or competencies and may be established for an entire course or for specific clinical activities. The objectives specify the acquisition of knowledge, development of values, and performance of psychomotor and technological skills.

The objectives for clinical practice should be communicated clearly to students, in written form, and understood by them. Similarly, the teacher has an important responsibility in discussing these outcomes and related clinical activities with agency personnel.

Teaching begins at the level of the learner. The teacher's goal, therefore, is to assess (1) the student's present level of knowledge and skill and (2) other characteristics that may influence achieving the objectives. In the first area of assessment, data are collected on whether the student possesses the prerequisite knowledge and skills for the clinical situation at hand and for completing the learning activities. This assessment is important so that students engage in learning activities that build on their present knowledge and skills. When students lack the prerequisites, then the instruction can remedy these and more efficiently move students forward in their learning. The second area of assessment relates to individual characteristics of students that may influence their learning and clinical performance, such as age, learning style, and cultural background.

Following the assessment of learner needs and characteristics, the teacher plans and then delivers the instruction. In planning the learning activities, the main considerations are the objectives and individual learner needs. Other factors that influence decisions on clinical activities include the philosophy and goals of the nursing program, characteristics of the clinical setting, and teacher availability to guide learners.

The next step in the process of clinical teaching is that of guiding learners to acquire essential knowledge, skills, and values for practice. In this process of guiding learners, the teacher needs to be skilled in (1) observing clinical performance, arriving at sound judgments about that performance, and planning additional learning activities if needed and (2) questioning learners without interrogation. Open-ended questions about students' thinking and the rationale they used for arriving at clinical decisions foster development of critical thinking skills, an important outcome of clinical practice.

The last component of the clinical teaching process is evaluation. Clinical evaluation serves two purposes: formative and summative. Through formative evaluation the teacher monitors student progress in meeting the clinical objectives and demonstrating competency in clinical practice. Clinical evaluation that is formative is not intended for grading purposes; instead, it is designed to diagnose learning needs as a basis for further instruction.

Summative evaluation, in contrast, takes place at the end of the learning period to ascertain if the objectives have been achieved and the competencies developed. It occurs at the completion of a course, an educational program, orientation, and other types of programs. This type of clinical evaluation determines what *has been* learned rather than what *can be* learned.

There are many clinical evaluation methods from which to choose: rating scale, checklist, anecdotal note, simulation, role play, media clip, problem-solving strategies, case study, written assignment, journal, portfolio, clinical conference, clinical examination, and self-evaluation. The objectives and competencies guide the teacher in selecting clinical evaluation methods. Many of these methods are discussed in greater depth in later chapters.

REFERENCES

Bondy, K. N., Jenkins, K., Seymour, L., Lancaster, R., & Ishee, J. (1997). The development and testing of a competency-focused psychiatric nursing clinical evaluation instrument. *Archives of Psychiatric Nursing, 11*(2), 66–73.

Borbasi, S. A., & Koop, A. (1994). The objective structured clinical examination: Its appreciation in nursing education. *Australian Journal of Advanced Nursing, 11*(3), 33–40.

Bott, P. A. (1996). *Testing and assessment in occupational and technical education*. Boston: Allyn & Bacon.

Brookfield, S. D. (1995). *Becoming a critically reflective teacher*. San Francisco: Jossey-Bass.

Brown, H. N., & Sorrell, J. M. (1993). Use of clinical journals to enhance critical thinking. *Nurse Educator, 18*(5), 16–19.

Callister, L. C. (1993). The use of student journals in nursing education: Making meaning out of clinical experience. *Journal of Nursing Education, 32*, 185–186.

Dunn, S. V., & Hansford, B. (1997). Undergraduate nursing students' perceptions of their clinical learning environment. *Journal of Advanced Nursing, 25*, 1299–1306.

Fothergill-Bourbonnais, F., & Higuchi, K. S. (1995). Selecting clinical learning experiences: An analysis of the factors involved. *Journal of Nursing Education, 34*, 37–41.

Gomez, D. A., Lobodzinski, S., & West, C. D. H. (1998). Evaluating clinical performance. In D. M. Billings & J. A. Halstead (Eds.), *Teaching in nursing* (pp. 407–422). Philadelphia: Saunders.

Gronlund, N. (1993). *How to make achievement tests and assessments* (5th ed.). Needham Heights, MA: Allyn & Bacon.

Hodges, H. F. (1996). Journal writing as a mode of thinking for RN-BSN students: A leveled approach to learning to listen to self and others. *Journal of Nursing Education, 35*, 137–141.

Hoff, P. S. (1995). Adult learning and the nurse. In B. Fuszard (Ed.), *Innovative teaching strategies in nursing* (2nd ed., pp. 3–8). Gaithersburg, MD: Aspen.

Krichbaum, K., Rowan, M., Duckett, L., Ryden, M. B., & Savik, K. (1994). The Clinical Evaluation Tool: A measure of the quality of clinical performance of baccalaureate nursing students. *Journal of Nursing Education, 33*, 395–404.

Mundt, M. H. (1997). A model for clinical learning experiences in integrated health care networks. *Journal of Nursing Education, 36*, 309–316.

Nitko, A. J. (1996). *Educational assessment of students* (2nd ed.). Englewood Cliffs, NJ: Prentice-Hall.

Norton, B. (1998). From teaching to learning: Theoretical foundations. In D. M. Billings & J. A. Halstead (Eds.), *Teaching in nursing* (pp. 211–245). Philadelphia: Saunders.

Oermann, M. H. (1997). Evaluating critical thinking in clinical practice. *Nurse Educator, 22*(5), 25–28.

———. (1998a). How to assess critical thinking in clinical practice. *Dimensions of Critical Care Nursing, 17,* 322–327.

———. (1998b). Professional reflection: Have you looked in the mirror lately? *Orthopaedic Nursing, 17*(4), 22–26.

Oermann, M. H., & Gaberson, K. B. (1998). *Evaluation and testing in nursing education.* New York: Springer.

Quinn, F. M. (1995). *The principles and practice of nurse education* (3rd ed.). London: Chapman & Hall.

Reilly, D. E., & Oermann, M. H. (1992). *Clinical teaching in nursing education.* New York: National League for Nursing.

Sedlak, C. A. (1992). Use of clinical logs by beginning nursing students and faculty to identify learning needs. *Journal of Nursing Education, 33,* 389–394.

———. (1997). Critical thinking of beginning baccalaureate nursing students during the first clinical nursing course. *Journal of Nursing Education, 36,* 11–18.

6

Ethical and Legal Issues in Clinical Teaching

Clinical teaching and learning take place in a social context. Teachers, students, staff members, and patients have roles, rights, and responsibilities that sometimes are in conflict. These conflicts create ethical and legal dilemmas for clinical teachers. This chapter discusses some ethical and legal issues related to clinical teaching and offers suggestions for preventing, minimizing, and managing these difficult situations.

ETHICAL ISSUES

Ethical standards make it possible for nurses, patients, teachers, and students to understand and respect each other. Contemporary bioethical standards include those related to respect for human dignity, autonomy, and freedom; beneficence; justice; veracity; privacy; and fidelity (de Tornyay, 1988; Husted & Husted, 1995; Oermann & Gaberson, 1998; Theis, 1988). These standards are important considerations for all parties involved in clinical teaching and learning.

Learners in a Service Setting

If the word *clinical* means "involving direct observation of the patient," most clinical activities must take place where patients are. Traditionally, learners encounter patients in health care service settings, such as acute care, extended care, and rehabilitation facilities. With the current focus on primary prevention, however, patients increasingly receive health care in home, community, and school environments (Stokes, 1998). Whatever the setting, patients are there to receive health care, staff members have the responsibility to provide care, and students are present to learn. Are these purposes always compatible?

Although it has been more than two decades since Corcoran (1977) raised ethical questions about the use of service settings for learning activities, those concerns are still valid. In the clinical setting, learners are nursing students or new staff members who are somewhat less skilled than experienced practitioners. Although their activities are observed and guided by clinical teachers, learners are not expected to provide cost-effective, efficient patient care services. On the other hand, patients expect quality service when they seek health care; providing learning opportunities for students usually is not a priority. The ethical standard of beneficence refers to the duty to help, to produce beneficial outcomes, or at least to do no harm (Husted & Husted, 1995). Is this standard violated when the learners' chief purpose for being in the clinical environment is to learn, not to give care?

Patients who encounter learners in clinical settings may feel exploited or fear invasion of their privacy; they may receive care that takes more time and creates more discomfort than if provided by expert practitioners. The presence of learners in a clinical setting also requires more time and energy of staff members, who usually are expected to give and receive reports from students, answer their questions, and demonstrate or help with patient care. These activities may divert staff members' attention from their primary responsibility for patient care, interfere with their efficient performance, and affect their satisfaction with their work (Corcoran, 1977; Infante, 1985).

Because achieving the desired outcomes of clinical teaching requires learning activities in real service settings, teachers must consider the rights and needs of learners, patients, and staff members when planning clinical learning activities. Corcoran (1977) suggested that the teacher is responsible for making the learning objectives clear to all involved persons and for ensuring that learning activities do not prevent achievement of service goals. Patients should receive adequate information about the presence of learners before giving their informed consent to participate in clinical learning activities. The teacher should assure the learners' preparation and readiness for clinical learning as well as his or her own presence and competence as an instructor, as discussed in Chapter 3.

Student-Faculty Relationships

RESPECT FOR PERSONS

As discussed in Chapter 1, an effective and beneficial relationship between clinical teacher and student is built on a base of mutual trust and respect. Although both parties are responsible for maintaining this relationship, the clinical teacher must initiate it by demonstrating trust and respect for students. A trusting, respectful relationship with students demonstrates the teacher's commitment to ethical values of respect for human dignity and autonomy (de Tornyay, 1988).

In a study by Theis (1988) of nursing students' perceptions of unethical teaching behaviors, 50% of the incidents described by students occurred in clinical settings, as compared with 39% in the classroom. Of the clinical incidents, 58% were classified as violations of respect for persons. Examples of such behavior included questioning and criticizing students in public areas, talking about a patient in the patient's presence, and allowing students to observe a catheterization without asking the patient's permission. As these examples illustrate, a clinical teacher's failure to model respect for patients also can be considered an unethical teaching behavior. Theis pointed out that in some instances, the teacher's behavior may have been misinterpreted by students. For example, while the student believed that the instructor failed to seek the patient's consent to the presence of observers, the instructor may have done so when the student was not present. However, if the teacher had obtained consent, pointing this out to the student would have prevented the misunderstanding as well as reinforced the ethical value of respect for patients (Theis, 1988).

FAIRNESS AND JUSTICE

The ethical standard of justice refers to fair treatment—judging each person's behavior by the same standards. Clinical teachers must evaluate each student's performance by the same standard. Students may perceive a clinical teacher's behavior as unfair when the teacher appears to favor some students by praising, supporting, and offering better learning opportunities to them more than others (Theis, 1988). Teachers who develop social relationships with some students are more likely to be perceived as unfair by other students. The teacher's relationships with students should be collegial and collaborative without being overly personal and social (Halstead, 1998b).

Students' Privacy Rights

When students have a succession of clinical instructors, it is common for the instructors to communicate information about student performance. Learning about the students' levels of performance in their previous clinical assignment helps the next instructor to anticipate their needs and to plan appropriate learning activities for them. Although students usually benefit when teachers share such information about their learning needs, personal information that students reveal in confidence should not be shared with other teachers. Additionally, when sharing information about students, teachers should focus on factual statements about performance without adding their personal judgments. Characterizing or labeling students is rarely helpful to the next instructor, and such behavior violates ethical standards of privacy as well as respect for individuals.

Competent Teaching

Applying the ethical standard of beneficence to teaching, students have a right to expect that their clinical teachers are competent, responsible, and knowledgeable (Theis, 1988). As discussed in Chapter 4, clinical competence, including expert knowledge and clinical skill, is an essential characteristic of effective clinical teachers. In addition, clinical teachers must be competent in (1) facilitating and supporting students in their learning activities, including planning assignments that help the students apply knowledge to practice, promoting student independence, and asking and answering questions; (2) evaluating student performance, including giving specific, timely feedback; and (3) communicating effectively with students, including developing collegial relationships with them (De Young, 1990; Reilly & Oermann, 1992; Stokes, 1998). Examples of unethical behavior related to clinical teacher competence include not being available for guidance in the clinical setting and demonstrating or directing a student to perform a skill in a manner that violated aseptic technique (Theis, 1988).

Academic Dishonesty

Although cheating and other forms of dishonest behavior are believed to be common in the classroom environment, academic dishonesty can occur in clinical settings as well. Academic dishonesty is defined as intentional participation in deceptive practices regarding the academic work of self or others. Dishonest acts include lying, cheating, plagiarizing, altering or forging records, falsely representing oneself, and knowingly assisting another person to commit a dishonest act (Gaberson, 1997).

Cheating is the use of unauthorized help in completing an academic assignment. An example of cheating is copying portions of a classmate's case study analysis and presenting the assignment as one's own work. Similarly, the student who asks a staff member's assistance to calculate a medication dose but tells the instructor that he or she did the work alone also is cheating (Gaberson, 1997).

Other examples of academic dishonesty in the clinical setting include:

- *Lying:* A student tells the instructor that she attempted a home visit to a patient but the patient was not at home. In fact, the student overslept and missed the scheduled time of the visit.
- *Plagiarism:* While preparing materials for a patient teaching project, a student paraphrases portions of a published teaching pamphlet without citing the source.
- *Altering a document:* A staff nurse orientee adds information to the documentation of nursing care for a patient on the previous day.
- *False representation:* As a family nurse practitioner student begins a physical examination, the patient addresses the student as "Doctor." The student continues with the examination and does not tell the patient that he is in fact a nurse.
- *Assisting another in a dishonest act:* Student A asks Student B to "cover" for her while she leaves the clinical agency to run a personal errand. The teacher asks Student B if he has seen Student A; Student B says that he thinks she has accompanied a patient to the physical therapy department.

While some of the previous examples may appear to be harmless or minor infractions, dishonest acts should be taken seriously because they can have harmful effects on patients, learners, faculty-student relationships, and the educational program. Clinical dishonesty can jeopardize patient safety if learners fail to report errors or do not receive adequate guidance because their competence is assumed. Mutual trust forms the basis for effective teacher-learner relationships, and academic dishonesty can damage a teacher's trust in students. Dishonesty that is ignored by teachers conveys the impression to students that this behavior is acceptable, and honest students resent teachers who fail to deal effectively with cheating. An educational program's reputation can be damaged when agency staff members discover clinical errors that have been concealed by students and not addressed by teachers; the result may be the loss of that agency for future clinical activities (Bradshaw & Lowenstein, 1990; Gaberson, 1997; Hoyer, Booth, Spelman, & Richardson, 1991).

Clinical academic dishonesty usually results from one or more of the following factors:

- *Competition.* Competition for good grades in clinical nursing courses may result from student misunderstanding of the evaluation framework. If students believe that a limited number of good grades is available, they may compete fiercely with their classmates. Competition may lead to deceptive acts in an attempt to earn higher grades than other students.
- *Emphasis on perfection.* Clinical teachers often communicate the expectation that good nurses do not make mistakes. Although nursing education attempts to prepare practitioners who will perform carefully and skillfully, a standard of perfection is unrealistic (Gaberson, 1997; Reilly & Oermann, 1992). Students naturally make mistakes in the process of learning new knowledge and skills, and punishment for mistakes, in the form of low grades or a negative performance evaluation, will not prevent these errors. In fact, it is the fear of punishment that often motivates students to conceal errors, and errors that are not reported are often harmful to patient safety.
- *Poor role modeling.* The influence of role models on behavior is strong. Nursing students and novice staff nurses who observe dishonest behavior of teachers and experienced staff members may emulate these examples, especially when the dishonest acts have gone unnoticed, unreported, or unpunished.
- *Impaired moral development.* Moral development is a socialization process in which nursing students learn to practice with integrity, according to the values of professional nursing. Commitment to these values and to the service of society obligates nursing faculty members to take responsibility for the moral development of their students. The nursing curriculum must reflect the values of the profession and should be structured to nurture the moral development of students, particularly if they enter nursing education with immature or undeveloped moral reasoning skills (Gaberson, 1997).

Clinical teachers can use a variety of approaches to discourage academic dishonesty. They should be exemplary role models of honest behavior for learners to emulate. They should acknowledge that mistakes occur in the learning process and create a learning climate that allows students to make mistakes in a safe environment with guidance and feedback for problem solving. However, students need reassurance that, if humanly possible, teachers will not allow them to make errors that would harm patients. Finally, each nursing education program should develop a policy that defines academic dishonesty and specifies appropriate penalties for violations. This policy should be communicated to all students, reviewed with them at regular intervals, and applied consistently and fairly to every violation (Gaberson, 1997).

When enforcing the academic integrity policy, it is important to apply ethical standards to protect the dignity and privacy of students. A public accusation of dishonesty that is found later to be ungrounded can damage a student's reputation. The teacher should speak with the student privately and calmly, describe the student's behavior and the teacher's interpretation of it, and provide the student with an opportunity to respond to the charge. It is essential to keep an open mind until all available evidence is evaluated because the student may be able to supply a reasonable explanation for the behavior that the teacher interpreted as cheating (Gaberson, 1997).

LEGAL ISSUES

It is beyond the scope of this book to discuss and interpret all federal, state, and local laws that have implications for clinical teaching and evaluation, and the authors are not qualified to give legal advice to clinical teachers regarding their practice. It is recommended that clinical teachers refer questions about the legal implications of policies and procedures to the legal counsel for the institution in which they are employed; concerns about a teacher's legal rights in a specific situation are best referred to the individual's attorney. However, this section of the chapter discusses common legal issues that often arise in the practice of clinical teaching.

Students With Disabilities

Two relatively recent federal laws have implications for the education of learners with disabilities. The Rehabilitation Act of 1973, Section 504, prohibits public postsecondary institutions that receive federal funding from denying access or participation to individuals with disabilities. The Americans with Disabilities Act (ADA) of 1990 guarantees persons with disabilities equal access to educational opportunities if they are otherwise qualified for admission (Halstead, 1998a). A qualified individual with a disability is one who has a physical or mental impairment that substantially limits one or more of that individual's major life activities. In nursing education programs, qualified individuals with disabilities are those who meet the essential requirements for participation, with or without modifications (Davidson, 1994).

A common goal of nursing education programs is to produce graduates who can function safely and competently in the roles for which they were prepared. For this reason, it is appropriate for those who make admission decisions to determine whether applicants could reasonably be expected to develop the necessary competence. The first step in this decision process is to define the essential functions necessary for participation in the program. Since nursing is a practice discipline, essential functions include cognitive, sensory, affective, and psychomotor performance requirements. It is recommended that such lists of essential functions be shared with applicants to nursing education programs to allow them to make initial judgments about their qualifications (Davidson, 1994).

Persons with disabilities who are admitted to nursing education programs are responsible for informing the institution of the disability and requesting reasonable accommodations (Letizia, 1995). Each nursing education program must determine on an individual basis whether the necessary modifications reasonably can be made. Reasonable accommodations for participating in clinical learning activities might include

- allowing additional time for a student with a qualified learning disability to complete an assignment (Letizia, 1995),
- allowing additional time to complete the program (Halstead, 1998a),
- scheduling clinical learning activities in facilities that are readily accessible to and usable by individuals who use wheelchairs or crutches, and
- providing the use of an amplified stethoscope for a student with a hearing impairment.

Reasonable accommodations do not include lowering academic standards or eliminating essential technical performance requirements. However, nurse educators need to distinguish essential from traditional functions by discussing such philosophical issues as whether individuals who will never practice bedside nursing in the conventional manner should be admitted to nursing education programs (Halstead, 1998a; Magilvy & Mitchell, 1995).

Due Process

Another legal issue related to clinical teaching is that of student rights to due process. In educational settings, due process requires that students be informed of the standards by which their performance will be judged, that they will receive timely feedback about their performance, and that they will have an opportunity to correct behavior that does not meet standards. In other words, learners have the right to be informed of their academic deficiencies, how those deficiencies will affect their academic progress, and what they need to do to correct the problem (Graveley & Stanley, 1993; Halstead, 1998b). Students who experience academic failure or dismissal from a nursing education program often appeal these decisions on the basis of denial of due process.

The 14th Amendment of the United States Constitution specifies that the state cannot deprive a person of life, liberty, or property without due process of law. With regard to the rights of students to due process, however, this constitutional protection extends only to those enrolled in public institutions. Students at private institutions instead may base a claim against the school on discrimination or contract law (Graveley & Stanley, 1993; Halstead, 1998b). For example, if a private school publishes a code of student rights and procedures for student grievances in its student handbook, those documents may be regarded as part of a contract between the school and the student. In paying and accepting tuition, the student and the school jointly agree to abide by this code of rights and set of procedures (Halstead, 1998b; Parrott, 1993; Reilly & Oermann, 1992). A student may sue on the basis of breach of contract if the school does not follow the stated due process procedures.

Courts hold different standards for due process based on whether it applies to academic or disciplinary decisions. Academic decisions include assigning a failing grade in a course, delaying progress, and dismissal from a program because of failure to maintain acceptable academic standing. The courts traditionally have been reluctant to intervene in academic decisions, believing that faculty are competent to judge student performance according to academic criteria or objectives (Parrott, 1993). Thus, academic due process is viewed by the courts as substantive due process, and the following procedures are generally sufficient:

- Students are informed in advance about the academic standards that will be used to judge their performance and about the process for appealing such decisions.
- Students are notified about the potential for academic failure well before grading decisions are made. Ideally, notification occurs orally and in writing, and the teacher and student work together to determine a plan for overcoming the deficiencies.
- Student performance is evaluated using the stated standards or criteria, and grades are assigned according to the stated policy.
- If a student believes that a grade or other academic decision is unfair, the stated appeal or grievance process is followed. Usually, the first level of appeal is to the teacher or group of faculty who assigned the grade. If the conflict is not resolved at that level, the student usually has the right of appeal to the administrator to whom the teacher reports. The next level of appeal usually is to a student standing committee or appeal panel of nursing faculty members. Finally, the student should have the right to appeal the decision to the highest level administrator in the nursing program.

Of course, if students exhaust every level of appeal and still are not sat-isfied with the outcome, they have the right to seek relief in the court sys-tem. It is important to note that the courts will allow such a lawsuit to go forward only if there is evidence that the student has first exhausted all internal school remedies. However, if the educational program faculty and administrators have followed substantive due process procedures as described above, it is unlikely that the academic decision will be reversed. If the student appeals to a court of law, the burden of proof that academic due process was denied rests with the student. With regard to due process for academic decisions, the key to resolving conflict and minimizing fac-ulty liability is in maintaining communication with students whose per-formance is not meeting standards (Halstead, 1998b).

Disciplinary decisions such as dismissal on the basis of misconduct or dishonesty require a higher level of due process, called procedural due process. Procedural due process guarantees the right to a hearing before dismissal. Components of disciplinary due process include the following:

- The student is provided with adequate written notice, including spe-cific details concerning the misconduct. For example, a notice may inform the student that she or he failed to attend a required clinical activity; that neither the faculty member nor nursing unit secretary was informed of the anticipated absence, in violation of school pol-icy on professional conduct; and that since this incident represented the third violation of professional conduct standards, the student would be dismissed from the program, according to the sanctions provided in the policy.
- The student is provided the opportunity for a fair, impartial hearing on the charges. The student has the right to speak on his or her own behalf, to present witnesses and evidence, and to question the other participants in the case (usually teachers and administrators). Using the example above, the student might present evidence that she did attempt to call the faculty member to report her absence; this evi-dence could include the date and time of the call, the name of the person with whom she spoke, and a copy of a telephone bill with the toll call charge. Although the student and the faculty member are entitled to the advice of legal counsel, neither attorney may ques-tion or cross-examine witnesses.

If the decision of the hearing panel is to uphold the dismissal, the stu-dent has the right to seek remedy from the court system if he or she believes that due process was not followed. However, in disciplinary cases, the burden of proof that due process was denied rests with the student.

Negligence, Liability, and Unsafe Clinical Practice

According to Lessner (1990), teachers and students are held to the same standards of care that a reasonably prudent person with the same level of education and experience would use in the same or similar circumstances. Thus, students are liable for their own actions as long as they are performing according to the usual standard of care for their education and experience, and they seek guidance when they are uncertain what to do. Teachers are not liable for negligent acts performed by their students as long as they have (1) selected appropriate learning activities based on objectives, (2) determined that students have prerequisite knowledge, skills, and attitudes necessary to complete their assignments, and (3) provided competent guidance. Therefore, it is not true that students practice under the faculty member's license. However, teachers are liable for their negligent actions if they make assignments that require more knowledge and skill than the learner has developed, or if they fail to guide student activities appropriately (Reilly & Oermann, 1992).

If a student demonstrates clinical performance that potentially is unsafe, the student and the teacher who made the assignment may be liable for any subsequent injury to the patient. However, since time for learning must precede time for evaluation, is it fair for the teacher to remove the student from the clinical area when to do so would prevent the student's access to learning opportunities for which he or she has paid tuition? In this case, denying access to clinical learning activities because of unsafe practice should not be considered an academic grading decision. Instead, it is an appropriate response to protecting the rights of patients to safe, competent care. The teacher's failure to take such protective action potentially places the teacher and the educational program at risk for liability (Parrott, 1993). Instead of denying the student access to all learning opportunities, removal from the clinical setting should be followed by a substitute assignment that would help the student to remove the deficiency in knowledge, skill, or attitude. For example, the student might be given a library assignment to acquire the information necessary to guide safe patient care, or an extra skills laboratory session could be arranged to allow more practice of psychomotor skills. A set of standards on safe clinical practice and a school policy that enforces the standards are helpful guides to faculty decision making and action while protecting student and faculty rights. Table 6.1 is an example of safe clinical practice standards, and Table 6.2 is an example of a policy that enforces these standards.

Table 6.1 Standards of Safe Clinical Practice

DUQUESNE UNIVERSITY
SCHOOL OF NURSING
BSN PROGRAM
STANDARDS OF SAFE CLINICAL PRACTICE

In all clinical situations, students are expected to demonstrate responsibility and accountability as professional nurses, with the ultimate goal being health promotion and prevention of harm to others. The School of Nursing believes that this goal will be attained if each student's daily clinical practice is guided by the Standards of Safe Clinical Practice.

Safe clinical performance always includes, but is not limited to, the following behaviors; therefore, I will:

1. Practice within boundaries of the nursing student role.
2. Comply with instructional policies and procedures on implementing nursing care.
3. Prepare for clinical assignments according to course requirements and as determined for the specific clinical setting.
4. Provide nursing care that may be required to promote health and prevent illness or further complications.
5. Demonstrate the application of previously learned skills and principles in providing nursing care.
6. Administer medications and/or treatments responsibly according to guidelines provided by the School of Nursing and agency.
7. Promptly report significant client information in a clear, accurate, and complete oral or written manner to the appropriate person(s).

Acknowledgment

I have read the Duquesne University School of Nursing Standards of Safe Clinical Practice. I understand that these standards are expectations that guide my clinical practice and will be incorporated into the evaluation of my clinical performance in all clinical courses. Failure to meet these standards may result in my removal from the clinical area, which may result in clinical failure.

_____

Signature and Date

Note: From Duquesne University School of Nursing, Pittsburgh, PA. Reprinted with permission.

Table 6.2 Policy on Safe Clinical Practice

DUQUESNE UNIVERSITY
SCHOOL OF NURSING
BSN PROGRAM
SAFE CLINICAL PRACTICE POLICY

POLICY: During enrollment in the Duquesne University School of Nursing BSN Program, all students, in all clinical activities, are expected to practice according to the Standards of Safe Clinical Practice.

Failure to abide by these standards will result in disciplinary action, which may include dismissal from the Nursing Program.

PROCEDURES: 1. Basic and Second Degree students will receive a copy of the Standards of Safe Clinical Practice at the beginning of N262, Health Promotion, or N205, Introduction to Professional Nursing. RN/BSN students will receive a copy of the Standards at the beginning of their first clinical course.
2. The Standards of Safe Clinical Practice will be reviewed with all students at the beginning of the clinical courses specified in 1. At that time, students will be required to sign a statement that they have read and understand the Standards. This statement will be kept during the student's enrollment in the BSN Program.
3. At the beginning of each subsequent academic year, the Standards of Safe Clinical Practice will be reviewed with students by the appropriate course facilitator.
4. Violation of these Standards will result in the following disciplinary action:
   a. First Violation
      1) Student will be given an immediate oral warning by the appropriate faculty member. The incident will be documented by the faculty member on the *Violation of Standards of Safe Clinical Practice* form. One copy of this form will be given to the student and one copy will be kept in the student's confidential record.
      2) At the discretion of the faculty member, the student may be required to leave the clinical

Table 6.2 *(continued)*

unit for the remainder of that day. The student may be given an alternative assignment.

3) If this violation is of a serious nature, it may be referred to the Associate Chair, BSN Program, and the Dean of Nursing for further disciplinary action as in b. and c., below.

b. Second Violation

1) The faculty member will document the incident on the *Violation of Safe Clinical Practice* form. Following discussion of the incident with the student, the faculty member will forward a copy of the form to the Associate Chair, BSN Program, for review and recommendation regarding further action.

2) The recommendation of the Associate Chair, BSN Program, will be forwarded to the Chair, BSN Program, for review and recommendation regarding reprimand or dismissal. If necessary, the Chair's recommendation will be forwarded to the Dean of the School of Nursing for final decision. This disciplinary action process will be documented and placed in the student's confidential record.

c. If the student has not been dismissed and remains in the Program following the above disciplinary action, any additional violation will be documented and referred as above to the Associate Chair, BSN program; the Chair, BSN Program; and the Dean of the School of Nursing for disciplinary action which may result in student dismissal from the Program.

d. The rights of students will be safeguarded as set forth in the Duquesne University *Code of Student Rights, Responsibilities, and Conduct* published in the current *University Student Handbook*.

Note. From Duquesne University School of Nursing, Pittsburgh, PA. Reprinted with permission.

Documentation and Record Keeping

Teachers should keep records of their evaluations of student clinical performance. These records may include anecdotal notes, summaries of faculty-student conferences, progress reports, and summative clinical evaluations. These records are helpful in documenting that students received feedback about their performance, areas of teacher concern, and information about student progress toward correcting deficiencies (Halstead, 1998b).

An anecdotal note is a narrative description of the observed behavior of the student, in relation to specific learning objectives. The note also may include the teacher's interpretation of the behavior, recorded separately from the description. Limiting the description and optional interpretation to a specified clinical objective avoids recording extraneous information, which is an ineffective use of the teacher's time. Anecdotal notes should record both positive and negative behaviors so as not to give the impression that the teacher is biased against the student. Students should review these notes and have an opportunity to comment on them; used in this way, anecdotal notes are an effective means of communicating formative evaluation information to students (Reilly & Oermann, 1992). Some sources recommend that both teacher and student sign the notes (Halstead, 1998b).

Writing anecdotal notes for every student, every day, is unnecessarily time-consuming. An effective, efficient approach might be to specify a minimum number of notes to be written for each student in relation to specified objectives (Reilly & Oermann, 1992). A student whose performance is either meritorious or cause for concern might prompt the instructor to write more numerous notes.

Records of student-teacher conferences likewise are summaries of discussions that focused on areas of concern, plans to address deficiencies, and progress toward correcting weaknesses. These conferences should take place in privacy and should address the teacher's responsibility to protect patient safety, concern about the student's clinical deficiencies, and a sincere desire to help the student to improve. During the conference, the student also has opportunities to clarify and respond to the teacher's feedback. At times, an objective third party such as a department chairperson or program director may be asked to participate in the conference in order to witness and clarify the comments of both teacher and student. The conference note should record the date, time, and place of the conference; the names and roles of participants; and a summary of the discussion, recommendations, and plans. The note may be signed only by the teacher or by all participants, according to institutional policy or guidelines (Halstead, 1998b).

Because they contain essentially formative evaluation information, anecdotal notes and conference notes should not be kept in the student's permanent record. Teachers should keep these records in their private files, taking appropriate precautions to ensure their security, until there is no reasonable expectation that they will be needed. In most cases, when the learner successfully completes the program or withdraws in good academic standing, these records can be discarded (again, taking appropriate security precautions). It is unlikely that successful learners will appeal favorable academic decisions. However, it is recommended that anecdotal records and conference notes be kept for longer periods when there is a chance that the learner may appeal the grade or other decision. The statute of limitations for such an appeal is a useful guide to deciding how long to keep those materials. It is recommended that teachers consult with legal counsel if there is a question as to institutional policy on retention of records.

SUMMARY

Because clinical teaching and learning take place in a social context, the rights of teachers, students, staff members, and patients sometimes are in conflict. These conflicts create legal and ethical dilemmas for clinical teachers. This chapter discussed some ethical and legal issues related to clinical teaching.

Ethical standards such as respect for human dignity, autonomy, and freedom; beneficence; justice; veracity; privacy; and fidelity are important considerations for all parties involved in clinical teaching and learning. Students must learn to apply these standards to nursing practice and teachers must apply them in their relationships with students as well as their teaching and evaluation responsibilities.

Specific ethical issues related to clinical teaching and learning include the presence of learners in a service setting, the need for faculty student relationships to be based on justice and respect for individuals, students' privacy rights, teaching competence, and academic dishonesty. Legal issues that have implications for clinical teaching and learning include educating students with disabilities, student rights to due process for academic and disciplinary decisions, standards of safe clinical practice, student and teacher negligence and liability, and documentation and record keeping regarding students' clinical performance.

Suggestions were offered for preventing, minimizing, and managing these difficult ethical and legal situations. Laws and institutional policies often provide guidelines for action in specific cases. However, these suggestions should not be construed as legal advice, and teachers are advised to seek legal counsel in regard to specific questions or problems.

REFERENCES

Bradshaw, M. J., & Lowenstein, A. J. (1990). Perspectives on academic dishonesty. *Nurse Educator, 15*(5), 10–15.

Corcoran, S. (1977). Should a service setting be used as a learning laboratory? An ethical question. *Nursing Outlook, 25,* 771–774.

Davidson, S. (1994). The Americans with Disabilities Act and essential functions in nursing programs. *Nurse Educator, 19*(2), 31–34.

de Tornyay, R. (1988). Ethical teaching behaviors. *Journal of Nursing Education, 27,* 101.

DeYoung, S. (1990). *Teaching nursing.* Redwood City, CA: Addison-Wesley.

Gaberson, K. B. (1997). Academic dishonesty. *Nursing Forum, 32*(3), 14–20.

Graveley, E. A., & Stanley, M. (1993). A clinical failure: What the courts tell us. *Journal of Nursing Education, 32,* 135–137.

Halstead, J. A. (1998a). Teaching students with special needs. In D. M. Billings & J. A. Halstead (Eds.), *Teaching in nursing: A guide for faculty* (pp. 57–66). Philadelphia: Saunders.

————. (1998b). The academic performance of students: Legal and ethical issues. In D. M. Billings & J. A. Halstead (Eds.), *Teaching in nursing: A guide for faculty* (pp. 35–56). Philadelphia: Saunders.

Hoyer, P. J., Booth, D., Spelman, M. R., & Richardson, C. E. (1991). Clinical cheating and moral development. *Nursing Outlook, 39,* 170–173.

Husted, G. L., & Husted, J. H. (1995). *Ethical decision making in nursing* (2nd ed.). St. Louis: Mosby.

Infante, M. S. (1985). *The clinical laboratory in nursing education* (2nd ed.). New York: Wiley.

Lessner, M. W. (1990). Avoiding student-faculty litigation. *Nurse Educator, 15*(6), 29–32.

Letizia, M. (1995). Issues in the postsecondary education of learning-disabled nursing students. *Nurse Educator, 20*(5), 18–22.

Magilvy, J. K., & Mitchell, A. C. (1995). Education of nursing students with special needs. *Journal of Nursing Education, 34,* 31–36.

Oermann, M. H., & Gaberson, K. B. (1998). *Evaluation and testing in nursing education.* New York: Springer.

Parrott, T. E. (1993). Dismissal for clinical deficiencies. *Nurse Educator, 18*(6), 14–17.

Reilly, D. E., & Oermann, M. H. (1992). *Clinical teaching in nursing education* (2nd ed.). New York: National League for Nursing.

Stokes, L. (1998). Teaching in clinical settings. In D. M. Billings & J. A. Halstead, (Eds.), *Teaching in nursing: A guide for faculty* (pp. 281–297). Philadelphia: Saunders.

Theis, E. C. (1988). Nursing students' perspectives of unethical teaching behaviors. *Journal of Nursing Education, 27,* 102–106.

7

Choosing Clinical Learning Assignments

One of the most important responsibilities of a clinical teacher is selecting clinical assignments that are related to objectives, appropriate to students' levels of knowledge and skill, and challenging enough to motivate learning. Although directing a learner to provide comprehensive nursing care to one or more patients is a typical clinical assignment, it is only one of many possible assignments, and not always the most appropriate choice. This chapter presents a framework for selecting clinical learning assignments and discusses several alternatives to the traditional total patient care assignment.

PATIENT CARE VERSUS LEARNING ACTIVITY

When planning assignments, clinical teachers typically speak of "selecting patients" for whom students will care. However, as discussed in Chapter 1, the primary role of the nursing student in the clinical area is that of learner, not nurse. While it is true that nursing students need contact with patients in order to apply classroom learning to clinical practice, caring for patients is not synonymous with learning. Nursing students are *learning to care* for patients; they are not nurses with *responsibility for patient care* (Infante, 1985). Providing patient care does not guarantee transfer of knowledge from the classroom to clinical practice; instead, it often reflects work requirements of the clinical agency (Karuhije, 1997).

Many faculty members assume that caring for patients always constitutes a clinical assignment for students on every level of the nursing education program. Even in their earliest clinical courses, nursing students typically have responsibility for patient care while learning basic psychomotor and communication skills. However, "beginning level nursing students are not prepared to care for clients in today's acute care setting and this should not be an expectation" (Fugate & Rebeschi, 1992, p. 14). This early responsibility for patient care often creates anxiety that interferes with learning (Fugate & Rebeschi, 1992; Infante, 1985).

As discussed in Chapter 2, changes in health care, technology, society, and education influence the competencies needed for professional nursing practice. Learning outcomes necessary for safe, competent nursing practice today include cognitive skills of problem solving, decision making, and critical thinking, in addition to technical proficiency. If nurse educators are to produce creative, independent, assertive, and decisive practitioners, they cannot assume that students will acquire these competencies through patient care assignments (Infante, 1985). To produce these outcomes, clinical teachers should choose clinical assignments from a variety of learning activities, including participation in patient care.

FACTORS AFFECTING SELECTION OF CLINICAL ASSIGNMENTS

The selection of learning activities within the context of the clinical teaching process is discussed in Chapter 5. Clinical activities help learners to apply knowledge to practice, develop skills, and cultivate professional values. Clinical assignments should be selected according to criteria such as the learning objectives of the clinical activity, needs of patients, availability and variety of learning opportunities in the clinical environment, and the needs, interests, and abilities of learners (Reilly & Oermann, 1992; Stokes, 1998).

Learning Objectives

The most important criterion for selection of clinical assignments usually is the desired learning outcome. The teacher should structure each clinical activity carefully in terms of the learning objectives, and each clinical activity should be an integral part of the course or educational program (Infante, 1985).

It is essential that the instructor, students, and staff members understand the goals of each clinical activity. Depending on the level of the learner, students may have difficulty envisioning how broad program outcomes or course objectives can be achieved in the context of a specific clinical environment. It is the instructor's role to translate these outcomes into specific clinical objectives and to select and structure learning activities so that they relate logically and sequentially to the goals (de Tornyay & Thompson, 1987; Infante, 1985; Reilly & Oermann, 1992).

Learner Characteristics

As discussed in Chapter 5, the learner's educational level or previous experience, aptitude for learning, learning style, and specific needs, interests, and abilities should also influence the selection of clinical assignments. The teacher must consider these individual differences; all learners do not have the same needs, so it is unreasonable to expect them to have the same learning assignments on any given day (Reilly & Oermann, 1992).

For example, Student A learns skills at a slower pace than other students at the same level. The instructor should plan assignments so that this student has many opportunities for repetition of skills with feedback. For example, if the objective is to learn the skills of medication administration, most students might be able to learn those skills in a reasonable amount of time in the context of providing care to one or more patients. Student A might learn more effectively with an assignment to administer all medications to a larger group of patients over a period of 1 day or more, without other patient care responsibilities. When the student has acquired the necessary level of skill, the next clinical assignment might be to administer medications while learning other aspects of care for one or more patients.

Students who are able to achieve the objectives of the essential curriculum (see Chapter 1) rather quickly might receive assignments from the enrichment curriculum that allow them to focus on their individual needs. For example, a student who is interested in perioperative nursing might be assigned to follow a patient through a surgical procedure, providing preoperative care, observing or participating in the surgery, assisting in immediate postoperative care in the Postanesthesia Care Unit, and presenting a plan of care for home care in a postclinical conference.

Needs of Patients

Patient needs and care requirements also should be considered when planning clinical assignments for students. In relation to the learning objective, will the nursing care activities present enough of a challenge to the learner? Are they too complex for the learner to manage?

Even if patients signed a consent for admission to the health care facility that included an agreement to the participation of learners in their care, their wishes regarding student assignment and those of their family members should be respected. At times of crisis, patients and family members may not wish to initiate a new nurse-patient relationship with a nursing student or new employee orientee. Nursing staff members who have provided care to these patients often can help the clinical teacher determine if student learning needs and specific patient and family needs both can be met through a particular clinical assignment.

Timing of Activities and Availability of Learning Opportunities

Since the purpose of clinical learning is to foster application of theory to practice, clinical learning activities should be related to what is being taught in the classroom. Ideally, clinical activities are scheduled concurrently with relevant classroom content so that learners can make immediate transfer and application of knowledge to nursing practice. However, there is little evidence of a relationship between clinical learning outcomes and the structure, timing, and organization of clinical learning activities (Dunn, Stockhausen, Thornton, & Barnard, 1995; Infante, 1985; Stokes, 1998).

The availability of learning opportunities to allow students to meet objectives often affects clinical assignments. The usual schedule of activities in the clinical facility may determine the optimum timing of learning activities. For example, if the learning objective for a new nursing student is "Identifies sources of information about patient needs from the health record," it would be difficult for students to gain access to patient records at the beginning or end of a shift. Thus, scheduling learners to arrive at the clinical site at mid-morning may allow better access to the resources necessary for learning (deTornyay & Thompson, 1987).

Some clinical settings, such as outpatient clinics and operating rooms, are available both to patients and students only on a daytime, Monday through Friday schedule. In other settings, however, scheduling clinical learning assignments during evening or night hours or on weekend days may offer students better opportunities to meet certain objectives. If the learning objective is "Implements health teaching for the parents of a premature or ill neonate," the best time for students to encounter parents may be during evening visiting hours or on weekends. Using these time periods for clinical activities also may avoid two or more groups of learners from different educational programs being in the same clinical area simultaneously, affecting the availability of learning opportunities.

Of course, planning learning activities at such times potentially may conflict with family, work, and other academic schedules and commitments for both teachers and students (deTornyay & Thompson, 1987; Dunn et al., 1995; Stokes, 1998). In some cases (for example, with the use of preceptors) it is not necessary for the teacher to be present in the clinical setting with learners, thereby allowing more flexible scheduling of clinical activities.

OPTIONS FOR LEARNING ASSIGNMENTS

The creative teacher may select clinical assignments from a wide variety of learning activities. Several options for making assignments are discussed below.

Teacher-Selected or Learner-Selected Assignments

While it is the teacher's responsibility to specify the learning objective, learners should have choices of learning activities that will help them achieve the objective. With learning outcomes such as assertiveness, creativity, independence, problem solving, and critical thinking, teachers must allow learners to participate actively in selecting their own clinical activities. Allowing learners to participate in selecting their own assignments also may reduce student anxiety.

Of course, the teacher should offer guidance in selecting appropriate learning activities through questions or comments that require students to evaluate their own needs, interests, and abilities. Sometimes teachers need to be more directive; a student may choose an assignment that clearly requires more knowledge or skill than the student has developed. In this case, the teacher must intervene to protect patient safety as well as to help the student make realistic plans to acquire the necessary knowledge and skill. Other students may choose "safe" assignments that do not challenge their abilities; the teacher's role is to support and encourage such students to take advantage of opportunities to achieve higher levels of knowledge and skill.

Skill Focus versus Total Care Focus

As previously discussed, the traditional clinical assignment for nursing students is to give total care to one or more patients. However, not all learning objectives require students to practice total patient care. For example, if the objective is "Assess patient and family preparation for postoperative recovery at home," the student does not have to provide total care to the postoperative patient in order to meet the objective. The student could meet the objective by interviewing the patient and family, review-ing the patient's records, and observing the patient's or family member's return demonstration of a dressing change. Additionally, total patient care is an integrative activity that can be accomplished effectively only when students are competent in performing the component skills (Infante, 1985).

All students do not need to be engaged in the same learning activities at the same time. Depending on their individual learning needs, some stu-dents might be engaged in activities that focus on developing a particular skill, while others could be practicing more integrative activities such as providing total patient care.

Student-Patient Ratio Options

Although the traditional clinical assignment takes the form of one student to one patient, there are other assignment options. These options are described and compared below:

- *One student/one patient.* One student is responsible for certain aspects of care or for comprehensive care for one or more patients. The stu-dent works alone to plan, implement, and evaluate nursing care (de Tornyay & Thompson, 1987; Fugate & Rebeschi, 1992; Stokes, 1998). This type of assignment is advantageous when the objective is to integrate many aspects of care after the student has learned the indi-vidual activities (Infante, 1985).
- *Multiple-student/one patient.* Two or more students are assigned to plan, implement, and evaluate care for one patient. Each learner has a defined role, and all collaborate to meet the learning objective. Various models of dual or multiple assignments exist. For example, three students would read the patient record, review the relevant pathophysiology, and collaborate on an assessment and plan of care. Student A reviews information concerning the patient's medications, administers and documents all scheduled and p.r.n. medications, and manages the intravenous infusions. Student B focuses on pro-viding and documenting all other aspects of patient care. Student C evaluates the effectiveness of the plan of care, assists with physical care when needed, interacts with the patient's family, and gives report to appropriate staff members. Members of the learning team can switch roles on subsequent days. This assignment strategy is particularly useful when patients have complex needs that are beyond the capability of one student, although it can be used in any setting with a large number of students and a low patient census. Other advantages include reducing student anxiety and teaching

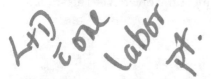

teamwork and collaborative learning (de Tornyay & Thompson, 1987; Fugate & Rebeschi, 1992; Stokes, 1998).

- *Multiple-student/patient aggregate.* A group of students is assigned to complete activities related to a community or population subgroup at risk for certain health problems. For example, a small group of students might be assigned to conduct a community assessment to identify an actual or potential health problem in the aggregate served by the clinical agency. Clinical activities would include interviewing community members and agency staff, identifying environmental and occupational health hazards, documenting the availability of social and health services, and performing selected physical assessments on a sample of the aggregate. The student group then would analyze the data and present a report to the agency staff and community members. Advantages of this assignment strategy include promoting a focus on community as client, teaching collaboration with other health care providers and community members, and reinforcement of group process (Doerr et al., 1998).

Management Activities

Some clinical assignments are chosen to enable learners to meet objectives related to nursing leadership, management and improvement of patient care, and meeting health care organizational goals. Undergraduate nursing students usually are introduced to concepts and skills of leadership and management in preparation for their future roles in complex health care systems. These students often benefit from clinical assignments that allow them to develop skill in planning and managing care for a group of patients. For example, a senior BSN student may enact the role of team leader for other nursing students who are assigned to provide total care for individual patients. The student-as-team-leader may receive report about the group of patients from agency staff, plan assignments for the other students, give a report to those students, supervise and coordinate work, and communicate patient information to staff members.

Master's and doctoral students may be preparing for management and administrative roles in health care organizations; their clinical activities might focus on enacting the roles of first-level or middle manager, patient care services administrator, or case manager (Oermann, 1997). New staff nurse employees usually need to be oriented to the role of charge nurse; assignments to help them learn the necessary knowledge, skills, and attitudes should include practice in this role. Often, such clinical assignments involve the participation of a preceptor (see the discussion of Models of Clinical Teaching in Chapter 4, and Chapter 14, Using Preceptors as Clinical Teachers).

Guided Observation

Observation is an important skill in nursing practice, and teachers should provide opportunities for learners to develop this skill systematically. Observing patients in order to collect data is a prerequisite to problem solving and clinical decision making. In order to make accurate and useful observations, the student must have knowledge of the phenomenon and the intellectual skill to observe it: the "what" and "how" of observation. As a clinical learning assignment, observation should not be combined with an assignment to provide care (Infante, 1985). If students do not have concurrent care responsibilities, they are free to choose the times and sometimes the locations of their observations. The focus should be on observing purposefully in order to meet a learning objective.

Observation also provides opportunities for students to learn through modeling. From observing another person performing a skill, the learner forms an image of how the behavior is to be performed, which serves as a guide to learning (Reilly & Oermann, 1992). For this reason, it is helpful to schedule learners to observe in a clinical setting before they are assigned to practice activities. However, scheduling an observation before the learner has acquired the prerequisite knowledge is unproductive; the student may not be able to make meaning out of what is observed.

Written observation guidelines can be used effectively to prepare learners for the activity and to guide their attention to important data during the observation itself. Table 7.1 is an example of an observation guide to prepare students for a group observation activity in an operating room. Note the explicit expectations that students will read, think critically, and anticipate what they will see, before the observation itself. The presence of an instructor or other resource person to answer questions and direct students' attention to pertinent items or activities also is helpful. Students may be asked to evaluate the observation activity by identifying learning outcomes, what they did and did not like about the activity, and the extent to which their preparation and the participation of the instructor was helpful. Table 7.2 is a sample evaluation tool for an observation activity.

SUMMARY

This chapter presented a framework for selecting clinical learning assignments. Clinical teachers should select clinical assignments that are related to objectives, appropriate to students' levels of knowledge and skill, and challenging enough to motivate learning. Providing comprehensive nursing care to one or more patients is a typical clinical assignment, but it is not always the most appropriate choice.

Table 7.1 Example of an Observation Guide

Operating Room Observation Guide

Purposes of the observation activity:

1. To gain an overview of perioperative nursing care in the intraoperative phase.

2. To observe application of principles of surgical asepsis in the operating room.

3. To distinguish among roles of various members of the surgical team.

General information:

You are expected to prepare for this observation and to complete an observation guide while you are observing the surgical procedure. Please read your medical-surgical nursing textbook for a general understanding of nursing roles in the intraoperative phase.

Bring this observation guide and a pen or pencil on the day of your observation. The guide will be collected and reviewed by the instructor at the end of the observation activity.

Most likely, you will observe either a coronary artery bypass graft or an aortic valve replacement. Please review the anatomy of the heart, specifically the coronary vessels and valves. In addition, read the following content in your medical-surgical nursing textbook: coronary artery disease; valvular heart disease (aortic stenosis).

After you have completed your reading assignment, attempt to answer the questions in the first section of the observation guide (Preparation of the Patient) related to preparations that take place before the patient comes to the operating room. Don't be afraid to make some educated guesses about the answers; we will discuss them and supply any missing information on the day of your observation.

Complete the remaining sections of the observation guide during your observation. The instructor will be available to guide the observation and to answer questions.

Operating Room Observation Guide
Preparation of the Patient

A. Who is responsible for obtaining the consent for the surgical procedure? Why?

B. Who identifies the patient when he or she is brought into the operating room? Why?

C. What other patient data should be reviewed by a nurse when the patient is brought to the operating room? Why?

(continued)

Table 7.1 (*continued*)

    D. Who transfers the patient from transport bed to the operating room bed? What safety precautions are taken during this procedure?

    E. What is the nurse's role during anesthesia induction?

    F. When is the patient positioned for the surgical procedure? Who does this? What safety precautions are taken? What special equipment may be used?

    G. What is the purpose of the preoperative skin preparation of the operative site? When is it done? What safety precautions are taken?

    H. What is the purpose of draping the patient and equipment? What factors determine the type of drape material used? What safety precautions are taken? Who does the draping? Why?

    I. What nursing diagnoses are commonly identified for patients in the immediate preoperative and early intraoperative phases?

Preparation of Personnel

    A. Apparel: Who is wearing what? What factors determine the selection of apparel? How and when do personnel don and remove apparel items? What personal protective equipment is used and why?

    B. Scrubbing: Which personnel scrub for the procedure? When?

    C. Gowning and gloving: What roles do the scrub person and the circulator play in these procedures?

Roles of Surgical Team Members

    A. Surgeons and assistants (surgical residents, interns, medical students)

    B. Nurses

    C. Anesthesia personnel

    D. Others (perfusion technologist, radiologic technologist, pathologist, etc.)

Maintenance of Aseptic Technique

    A. Movement of personnel

    B. Sterile areas/items

    C. Nonsterile areas/items

    D. Handling of sterile items

Table 7.1 *(continued)*

Equipment

    A. Lighting: Who positions it? How? When?

    B. Monitoring: What monitors are used? Who is responsible for setting up and watching this equipment?

    C. Blood/other fluid infusion: Who is responsible for setting up and monitoring this equipment?

    D. Electrocautery: What is this equipment used for? Who is responsible for it? What safety precautions are taken?

    E. Suction: What is this equipment used for? Who is responsible for setting up and monitoring it?

    F. Smoke evacuator: What is this equipment used for? Who is responsible for setting up and using it?

    G. Patient heating/cooling equipment: What is this equipment used for? Who is responsible for setting up and monitoring it?

    H. Other equipment:

Intraoperative and Early Postoperative Period Nursing Diagnoses

    A. What nursing diagnoses are likely to be identified for this patient in the intraoperative and early postoperative periods?

Clinical teachers typically speak of "selecting patients" for clinical assignments. However, the primary role of the nursing student in the clinical area is that of learner, not nurse. Caring for patients is not synonymous with learning. Nursing students are *learning to care* for patients; they are not nurses with *responsibility for patient care*. In fact, early responsibility for patient care often creates anxiety that interferes with learning.

Factors affecting the selection of clinical assignments include the learning objectives of the clinical activity, needs of patients, availability and variety of learning opportunities in the clinical environment, and the needs, interests, and abilities of learners. The most important criterion for selection of clinical assignments usually is the learning objective. Each clinical activity should be an integral part of the course or educational program, and it is essential that the instructor, students, and staff members understand the goals of each clinical activity. Learning activities are selected and structured so that they relate logically and sequentially to the objective.

Individual learner characteristics such as educational level, previous experience, aptitude for learning, learning style, and specific needs, interests, and abilities should also influence the selection of clinical assignments.

Table 7.2 Example of Student Evaluation of a Guided Observation Activity

Student Evaluation of OR Observation

1. To what extent did you prepare for this learning activity?
   - _____ 4. I completed all assigned readings and attempted answers to all questions on the first section of the observation guide.
   - _____ 3. I completed all assigned readings and attempted to answer some of the observation guide questions.
   - _____ 2. I completed some of the assigned readings and attempted to answer some of the observation guide questions.
   - _____ 1. I didn't do any reading but I tried to answer some of the observation guide questions before I came to the OR.
   - _____ 0. I didn't do any reading and I didn't answer any observation guide questions before I came to the OR.

2. How would you rate the overall value of this learning activity?
   - _____ 4. It was excellent; I learned a great deal.
   - _____ 3. It was very good; I learned more than I expected to.
   - _____ 2. It was good; I learned about as much as I expected to.
   - _____ 1. It was fair; I didn't learn as much as I expected to.
   - _____ 0. It was poor; I didn't learn anything of value.

3. How would you rate the value of the observation guide in helping you to prepare for and participate in the observation?
   - _____ 4. Extremely helpful in focusing my attention on significant aspects of perioperative nursing care.
   - _____ 3. Very helpful in guiding me to observe activities in the OR.
   - _____ 2. Helpful in guiding my observations, but at times distracted my attention from what I wanted to watch.
   - _____ 1. Only a little helpful; it seemed like a lot of work for little benefit.
   - _____ 0. Not at all helpful; it distracted me more than it helped me to observe what was going on in the OR.

4. How would you rate the helpfulness of the instructor who guided your OR observation?
   - _____ 4. Excellent; helped me to analyze, synthesize, and evaluate the activities I observed.

Table 7.2 *(continued)*

_____ 3. Very good; answered my questions and focused my attention on important activities.

_____ 2. Good; was able to answer some questions, attempted to make the activity meaningful to me.

_____ 1. Fair; I probably could have learned as much without an instructor present.

_____ 0. Poor; distracted me or interfered with my learning; I could have learned more without an instructor present.

5. What was the most meaningful part of this learning activity for you? What was the most important or surprising thing you learned?

6. What was the least meaningful part of this observation activity? If there is something that you would change, suggest what would make it better.

All learners do not have the same needs, so it is unreasonable to expect them to have the same learning assignments on any given day. Students who are able to achieve the objectives of the essential curriculum quickly might receive assignments from the enrichment curriculum that allow them to focus on their individual needs.

Patient needs and care requirements also should be considered when planning clinical assignments. The nursing care activities required by a patient may not present enough of a challenge to one learner or be too complex for another. Patient wishes regarding student assignment should be respected. Nursing staff members who have provided care to these patients often can help the clinical teacher determine if student learning needs and specific patient and family needs both can be met through a particular clinical assignment.

Another factor affecting the selection of clinical assignments is the timing and availability of learning opportunities. Ideally, clinical learning activities are scheduled concurrently with relevant classroom content so that learners can apply knowledge to nursing practice immediately. The usual schedule of activities in the clinical facility may determine the optimum timing of learning activities. Some clinical settings are available both to patients and students only at certain times. In other settings, however, scheduling clinical learning assignments during evening or night hours or on weekends provides better opportunities to meet objectives.

Alternatives for making clinical assignments include selection by teacher or learner, focus on particular skills or integrative patient care, various student-patient ratio options, management activities, and guided observation. Advantages and drawbacks of each alternative were discussed.

REFERENCES

de Tornyay, R., & Thompson, M. A. (1987). *Strategies for teaching nursing.* New York: Wiley.

Doerr, B., Sheil, E., Baisch, M. J., Forbes, S., Howe, C J., Johnson, M., & Vogtsberger, C. (1998). Beyond community assessment into the real world of learning aggregate practice. *Nursing and Health Care Perspectives, 19,* 214–219.

Dunn, S. V., Stockhausen, L., Thornton, R., & Barnard, A. (1995). The relationship between clinical education format and selected student learning outcomes. *Journal of Nursing Education, 34,* 16–24.

Fugate, T., & Rebeschi, L. M. (1992). Dual assignment: An alternative clinical teaching strategy. *Nurse Educator, 17*(6), 14–16.

Infante, M. S. (1985). *The clinical laboratory in nursing education* (2nd ed.). New York: Wiley.

Karuhije, H. F. (1997). Classroom and clinical teaching in nursing: Delineating differences. *Nursing Forum, 32*(2), 5–12.

Oermann, M. H. (1997). *Professional nursing practice.* Stamford, CT: Appleton & Lange.

Reilly, D. E., & Oermann, M. H. (1992). *Clinical teaching in nursing education* (2nd ed.). New York: National League for Nursing.

Stokes, L. (1998). Teaching in clinical settings. In D. M. Billings & J. A. Halstead (Eds.), *Teaching in nursing: A guide for faculty* (pp. 281–297). Philadelphia: Saunders.

8

Self-Directed Learning Activities

Many clinical objectives and competencies may be met by the students themselves through self-directed learning activities. These activities may involve instructional media, such as videotapes; multimedia, including computer-assisted instruction, interactive videodisc, CD-ROM, virtual reality, and the Internet; modules; and independent study.

There is a wide range of individual differences among students. Some students enter a clinical course with extensive knowledge and skills, whereas others may lack the prerequisite behaviors for engaging in the learning activities. Differences in learning styles, preferences for teaching methods, cultural backgrounds, and pace of learning all suggest a need for self-directed activities that reflect these individual variations among learners. With these activities, the responsibility for learning rests with the student.

There are varied types of self-directed activities for use in clinical teaching. Many of these activities are based on multimedia and instructional technology, whereas others, such as modules, may or may not use media. Self-directed activities may be required for completion by all students to meet the clinical objectives or for use by individual students for reinforcement of learning, continued practice of skills, and remedial instruction. Chapter 8 reviews self-directed learning activities appropriate for clinical teaching. The reader should recognize, however, that the activities involving multimedia are changing rapidly, and new technologies are continually being introduced for teaching and learning in clinical practice.

USING SELF-DIRECTED LEARNING ACTIVITIES

Self-directed learning activities are what the term suggests—activities directed by the students themselves. While planned by the teacher as part of the clinical activities, or recommended to meet specific learning needs, self-directed activities are intended for completion by the students on their own. These activities are typically self-contained units that students complete independently, often in a setting of their choice, and according to their own time frame. Computer-assisted instruction, for instance, may be completed in a learning laboratory or at home at a time convenient for the student. Learners may move through the instruction at a fast or slow pace depending on their learning needs and may repeat content and activities until competency is achieved. Many self-directed activities also include pre- and posttests for students to evaluate their own progress and learning at the end of the instruction.

Self-directed activities may be planned for completion by all students to meet certain clinical objectives or by students on an individual basis to reflect their particular learning needs. For some clinical courses and experiences, all students may be required to complete self-directed activities as a means of acquiring essential knowledge for practice and developing competencies associated with the clinical experience. These activities, then, would be integrated in the clinical course during its development.

When students lack prerequisite knowledge and skills, or when remedial instruction is warranted for some students but not others, self-directed activities provide a means of meeting these learning needs without requiring all students to complete the same learning activities. In these instances, the self-directed activities assist individual students in gaining knowledge and skills they need for practice. Self-directed activities, therefore, are an important adjunct to clinical teaching.

Along with allowing students to learn in a setting of their choice and at a time convenient for them, self-directed activities encourage them to assume responsibility for their own learning, an important outcome of nursing programs. The student becomes a self-learner, using and producing information for learning, rather than receiving it from the teacher (Hedberg, Brown, & Arrighi, 1997). Although beneficial for students, self-directed learning requires their commitment and motivation. The teacher may plan strategies, such as periodic quizzes, to monitor student progress in completing the learning activities, provide feedback, and assist students in developing their self-discipline. In some courses the faculty may establish time frames for completion of certain activities to better monitor progress and assure completion by the end of the course or clinical experience.

Using Self-Directed Activities for Cognitive Skill Development

Self-directed activities that depict clinical situations and patient care scenarios are particularly effective for promoting problem-solving, decision-making, and critical thinking skills. After viewing the clinical situation presented in the media or multimedia, students may be asked to

- identify the problems and issues to be solved and provide a supporting rationale
- identify alternate problems that might be possible in the clinical situation
- differentiate relevant and irrelevant information
- develop careful and pointed questions to clarify the problems and issues further
- identify additional data needed for decision making
- identify multiple approaches for solving the clinical problems and issues they identified, alternate approaches possible, and advantages and disadvantages of each
- compare varied decisions possible in a situation and outcomes
- decide on the approach they would use, or decision they would make, and provide a rationale underlying their thinking
- work backwards from the desired outcome to develop a plan for solving the problem (Nitko, 1996, p. 189)
- examine how key concepts and theories apply to the clinical situation depicted in the media or multimedia
- analyze the clinical scenario using theories described in class, in readings, and through other learning activities as a way of transferring learning to clinical practice
- identify assumptions made and how these influenced thinking
- articulate different points of view (Oermann & Gaberson, 1998).

PLANNING SELF-DIRECTED ACTIVITIES

While self-directed activities are completed by students themselves, the teacher, nevertheless, is responsible for planning those activities as part of the clinical experience or recommending them for students to meet individual learning needs. Self-directed learning activities, similar to other types of clinical activities, should be consistent with the clinical objectives. The main reason for their use in a clinical course is their potential to assist students in achieving certain outcomes.

In planning self-directed activities, the teacher should consider the resources needed for their implementation. These resources include costs for developing materials, purchasing commercially available materials, and supporting software and hardware; equipment needed; space, such as a computer laboratory; other requirements associated with a particular technology; and resources needed by students, such as Internet access. The time required for completion is another consideration in planning these activities for a course. Monitor the time students take for each activity so this information is available for planning at a later time.

One way of assuring effective planning and use of self-directed activities within a clinical course is to follow the acronym PLAN:

Plan activities that assist students in meeting the clinical objectives and/or individual learning needs.

Link these activities with the resources of the nursing program and those needed by students.

Assess prerequisite knowledge and skills for initiating the self-directed activities, students' progress as they complete them, and learning outcomes.

Never assume that students will learn at the same rate and in the same way; instead allow for individualization in types of learning activities, rates of learning, and outcomes.

When incorporating self-directed activities in clinical courses, students should have directions as to which activities to complete, how these activities promote achievement of the objectives, when the activities should be completed, and how they will be evaluated, if at all.

TYPES OF SELF-DIRECTED LEARNING ACTIVITIES

It is beyond the scope of this chapter to describe in detail all of the self-directed activities available for clinical teaching, particularly when considering the rapid growth of computer technology. While many self-directed methods are reviewed, they do not represent an exhaustive list and instead present a sampling of these activities and how they might be used in clinical teaching. In the chapter, self-directed activities are categorized as instructional media, such as videotapes; multimedia, including computer-assisted instruction, interactive videodisc, CD-ROM, virtual reality, and the Internet; modules; and independent study. There are different ways of grouping these methods for presentation in the chapter; this categorization represents only one way. The reader also should recognize that many of the activities use more than one method; for instance, modules typically incorporate multimedia.

Instructional Media

Instructional media and multimedia promote learning through different senses, making it easier to comprehend difficult concepts. Media that depict patient care scenarios help students understand how concepts and theories are used in practice and give them an idea of what a clinical situation is like. This vicarious experience prepares learners for the reality of clinical practice. Another important use of media in clinical teaching is the ability to present clinical situations involving ethical dilemmas and value conflicts for students to analyze. In this way students may gain experience in analyzing and responding to an ethical dilemma before encountering it in actual practice. Media for this purpose also provide a means for students to examine their own values that may influence the care of patients.

Media are effective for showing clinical situations that would normally be inaccessible to students, close-up pictures, and procedures. With technological skills, media provide a way of demonstrating the use of equipment and how to carry out a procedure in the clinical setting, emphasizing critical elements of performance.

There is a wide range of print and nonprint media available for clinical teaching (see Table 8.1). Research in nursing education suggests that media and multimedia are effective for acquiring new knowledge, learning problem solving, developing clinical skills, and promoting value development (Oermann, 1990).

Multimedia

Multimedia include computer-assisted instruction, interactive videodisc, CD-ROM, virtual reality, and the Internet. Multimedia are the combination of video, audio, text, and graphics that are presented using computer technology (Zwirn, 1998). Riley (1996) referred to these as computer-based educational activities. Multimedia, similar to media, may be used by all students to meet clinical learning outcomes or by individual students. A key concept of multimedia is the interaction between the computer program and the learner. By being interactive, the multimedia create an environment in which students are able to branch through the program based on their responses to questions raised about the content (Falk & Carlson, 1995).

Prior to using any multimedia for clinical teaching, the teacher should evaluate its content, including accuracy, organization, clarity in presenting the content, and comprehensiveness; relevance to the clinical course and clinical learning outcomes; usefulness for meeting individual student needs; currency in terms of clinical practice; extent of interaction between student and multimedia; cost; and resources needed for effective implementation (see Table 8.2). One other aspect of this evaluation relates to the

Table 8.1 Types of Instructional Media

Print

- Book
- Brochure and pamphlet
- Handout, diagram, and other types of written materials
- Study guide
- Workbook

Nonprint

- Audiotape
- CD-ROM
- Computer and related technology
- Film
- Model
- Overhead transparency
- Photograph
- Real object
- Slide
- Television
- Videodisc
- Videotape

appropriateness of the content for the clinical setting; with some multimedia, students may need to adapt interventions and procedures to their own clinical settings.

COMPUTER-ASSISTED INSTRUCTION

Computer-assisted instruction (CAI) uses the computer to guide learning; it provides instruction through the interaction of the student and the computer. CAI may be completed by a student individually with the computer or via a computer network in a learning resource center. It may be used to present new content important for clinical practice, to promote application of concepts and theories to simulated clinical situations, as a review prior to clinical practice, and to provide remedial instruction for individual students. While CAI may include a description of a clinical situation and illustrations of it, it does not have the sound and video images of interactive

Table 8.2 Evaluation of Multimedia for Clinical Teaching

Are the multimedia:

- Relevant to the clinical course? Clinical learning outcomes? Clinical settings where students have practice?
- Useful for meeting individual student needs?
- Able to be modified or adapted to better meet the objectives and learner needs?
- Of high technical quality (e.g., color, graphics, sounds, etc.)?

Is the content:

- Accurate?
- Organized logically?
- Presented clearly?
- Comprehensive?
- In sufficient depth for clinical course and learners?
- Up-to-date?

Does the instruction:

- Provide for interaction with the student?
- Give immediate feedback and reinforcement?
- Maintain student interest?
- Allow for entering and exiting the program as needed?
- Adapt for individual student needs?

Is the cost worth the investment?

Are there sufficient resources for implementation?

---

videodiscs. Nevertheless, it provides practice in applying theory to clinical situations and experiencing, at least hypothetically, a situation before encountering it in clinical practice.

CAI is often developed in the form of modules for ease of student use in directing their own learning. Gee, Peterson, Martin, and Reeve (1998) described the development of a CAI module for teaching clinical pharmacology to nursing students. The CAI module consisted of (1) objectives, (2) an introduction and review of relevant disease states, (3) a detailed discussion of each drug classification useful in treating different patient conditions, (4) guidelines for using drugs for managing these conditions, and (5) multiple-choice questions with explanations for both correct and incorrect answers for students to monitor their progress.

CAI typically incorporates questions for feedback to students, indicating which answers and decisions are correct or incorrect and why. The questions and answers also provide reinforcement for learning as students progress through the instruction. With CAI, students are able to pace themselves and repeat instruction as needed. CAI also has been found to decrease instructional time (Riley, 1996).

There are different types of CAI:

- *Drill and practice* allows the students to practice previously learned content by asking questions about the content and having students respond to them. The program provides immediate feedback on the accuracy of these answers. Drill and practice CAIs are often used for teaching factual information such as definitions of medical terms and calculations of dosages of medications.
- *Tutorials* provide more feedback during the instruction than drill and practice. Tutorials using branching techniques allow the students to move forward to learn new content or backward if remedial instruction is still needed. For clinical teaching, tutorials may be used to present new content for practice or for remedial instruction.
- *Simulations* present a real-life situation for analysis and decision making. With a simulation, the students make a series of clinical decisions similar to those needed in actual practice and receive immediate feedback on them. With some simulations the learners' decisions influence subsequent information presented. CAI simulations are particularly appropriate for gaining practice in analyzing client data, identifying problems and possible approaches to use, evaluating clinical situations, developing critical thinking skills, and making mistakes without affecting an actual patient (Reilly & Oermann, 1992; Riley, 1996; Zwirn, 1998).

While CAI programs have been used most frequently in nursing education programs, they also are useful for staff development and continuing education (Adsit, 1996; Davis, 1998; Edwards, 1995) and for teaching patients and families.

INTERACTIVE VIDEODISC INSTRUCTION

Interactive videodisc instruction (IVDI) is a type of CAI that combines a computer program with video images and sound from a laser disk (DeAmicis, 1997). In IVDI the computer augments the video display by (1) providing for interaction between the student and computer, making it easier to clarify difficult concepts and repeat instruction when unsure; (2) integrating questions for feedback and techniques for reinforcement of learning; and (3) including pre- and posttests for monitoring student progress.

IVDI allows for visualization of a clinical practice situation, creating real-life simulations for students to identify data to be collected, analyze data, plan care, select interventions, and evaluate changes in client conditions, all with immediate feedback from the computer. For this reason, IVDI is an important teaching method for promoting problem-solving, decision-making, and critical thinking skills. The IVDI series on leadership and management by FITNE, Inc. includes "think about" questions for discussion and case studies that portray problems often faced by nurse managers and supervisors. The case studies include questions for analysis, problem solving, and application of newly learned content (Shockley & Graveley, 1998).

IVDI also is valuable in teaching psychomotor skills in that students may progress through the program at their own pace, stopping when needed, then practice the skills in the learning laboratory. For instance, students may complete an IVDI on intravenous therapy, then practice in the learning laboratory assembling an IV, regulating the flow, and documenting it. Subsequent IVDI might include different patient scenarios involving intravenous therapy to expand on this learning and develop decision-making skills. DeAmicis (1997) compared the effectiveness of IVDI with traditional lecture and demonstration for teaching IV skills to baccalaureate nursing students. There was no significant difference between the two groups in ability to perform this skill. DeAmicis concluded that IVDI was an effective method for self-paced and independent learning of a psychomotor skill, consistent with earlier studies. Students may be less anxious performing a new skill in clinical practice when they have had prior experience with IVDI (Riley, 1996).

IVDI allows students to experiment and explore different decisions possible in a situation, gives immediate feedback on decisions made, and encourages students to evaluate their own clinical judgment skills. Not all students, though, learn at the same level with IVDI. Yoder (1994) found that students who preferred to learn by active experimenting achieved at a higher level with IVDI than students who preferred to learn by reflective observing.

CD-ROM

CD-ROMs also may be used for self-directed learning activities. For instance, there are CD-ROM programs for teaching basic skills such as blood pressure measurement, for teaching physical assessment, on pharmacology, and on care of patients with varied health problems. Simulations are available on CD-ROM that teach new clinical content and include scenarios for analysis and problem solving.

CD-ROMs often incorporate graphics, animation, photographs, and video segments. Ludy (1998) described patient simulation software by SimBioSys that provides an overview of the principles and practices of pulmonary function testing on a single CD-ROM. The CD-ROM includes hypertext-linked sections of technical data for performing and understanding pulmonary function tests, vocabulary words with linked definitions, examples of pulmonary function test tracings, links to explanations of more complex tests, and case studies for students to analyze.

VIRTUAL REALITY

Virtual reality is the display of scenes representing reality and control of these by the learner through use of gloves, joysticks, and helmets that sense the learner's movements (Gayeski, 1993). Virtual reality provides a three-dimensional image that is interactive. Virtual anatomical dissections and virtual reality applications for developing surgical and other types of skills and learning how to treat patients with different conditions are available already. Virtual reality simulators, though, are expensive, and users may suffer from motion sickness (Strauss, 1995). As this technology develops, teachers should familiarize themselves with available products. Virtual reality has much potential to expand the faculty's ideas of clinical practice (Carlton, 1996).

WORLD WIDE WEB AND THE INTERNET

The World Wide Web, a core part of the Internet, is a multimedia platform for accessing information that is organized in relationship to other information, enabling the student to retrieve it quickly and easily through different paths. The Web gives learners access to large databases, enables them to find answers to questions about patient problems and clinical situations, and allows students to select pathways through this information that are appropriate for their own learning needs and interests.

Khan (1997) defined Web-based instruction as an innovative approach for delivering instruction to a remote audience using the Web. The Web provides access to instructional resources from a distance and makes active learning possible. Illustrations, photos, x-rays, and film clips available on the Web may be integrated easily into clinical teaching. Thomson (1998) described how to develop a multimedia presentation on anatomy and physiology from Internet resources for teaching nursing students.

The Web relies on the use of hypertext, a multidimensional pathway linking words by associations (Gillham, 1998). A major advantage of hypertext for nursing education is that it allows for rapid navigation through large quantities of information (Gillham, 1998, p. 95). Given suitable computer and database access, students and nurses in practice can quickly retrieve information and gather possible answers to questions raised about patient care. Bridges and Thede (1996) cautioned that information on the World Wide Web needs to be evaluated by the user in terms of believability, reliability of the author, evidence provided for verifying the information, support for the author's claims, whether the information is logical, and its timeliness.

The Internet has opened many opportunities for self-directed activities to support clinical learning. Students may communicate with each other in the clinical group and with the teacher through electronic mail and may discuss clinical issues in chat groups set up by the faculty member. Students may be directed to Web sites related to the clinical objectives or to explore specific clinical issues faced in their practice. In the beginning of a clinical course, for example, students may explore sites relevant to the area of clinical practice, such as oncology nursing, and evaluate each site for its usefulness in caring for these patients, in patient education, or for their own learning. Rather than reading print materials to answer questions about clinical practice, students may find these answers on the Web, linking to different sites based on their learning needs and interests.

Faculty may develop case studies for student analysis and set up conferences and chat rooms where students and faculty can discuss the case studies further (Carlton, Ryan, & Siktberg, 1998). If resources are available, self-directed activities that are Web-based are limited only by the teacher's creativity and willingness to explore new technologies.

In using the Internet for teaching, McGonigle and Mastrian (1998) identified steps to create cyberspace quests or scavenger hunts. These steps are adapted for designing effective clinical learning activities that are Web-based:

1. Identify the goals for the self-directed activity on the Web, relate the activity to the clinical objectives, or determine how this Web-based activity will expand students' understanding of patient care and typical problems faced by patients in the clinical setting.
2. Identify the information about clinical practice that students are seeking on the Web. Describe this information in specific terms so students know exactly what they are looking for as they complete these Web-based activities. McGonigle and Mastrian (1998) recommended that the teacher seek and acquire the uniform resource locators, keep notes on the pathways used to get to the information, and develop related instruction and a tutorial for students (p. 83). While paths may be suggested for students, the teacher should realize that students will follow their own paths to find the information.
3. Another option is to design the learning activities by directing students to a particular site and planning activities for completion at

that site. For instance, students might be directed to Virtual Hospital at http://vh.radiology.uiowa.edu and asked to (a) locate information they could use in teaching their patients and (b) adapt this information to meet the learning needs of a patient for whom they have recently cared.

4. Identify completion dates for these learning activities and decide how students will submit them to faculty, for example, at the course Web page or via electronic mail.
5. Create orientation materials, instructions for students, and a tutorial (McGonigle & Mastrian, 1998).
6. Before using these Web-based activities, pilot them, keeping track of the time and ease for their completion.
7. Evaluate the effectiveness of the Web-based activities for obtaining the information and meeting the related clinical objectives, student ease in searching and navigating the Internet, the time required, and any problems encountered by students in completing these self-directed activities. This evaluation then provides a basis for revising the learning activities for subsequent use.

OTHER COMPUTER TECHNOLOGIES FOR SELF-DIRECTED LEARNING

There are many other computer technologies being developed that support clinical teaching and may be used for self-directed learning activities. For example, with distance education students can receive instruction at a location different from the teacher. Distance education uses a variety of strategies to connect students and faculty who otherwise could not meet because of time or distance (Billings, 1996; Clark, 1998). These strategies include print materials exchanged through the mail, such as self-paced modules on clinical concepts sent to students for their completion; two-way audio and audioconferencing using telephones to link the teacher with students in their homes or clinical facilities (Van Dusen, 1997); videoconferencing or interactive television, in which "classes are transmitted to distance sites by telephone, cable, satellite, or microwave" (Billings, 1996, p. 211); and instruction delivered by computer. A major advantage of distance education for clinical teaching is connecting learners with faculty and clinicians at different sites who are experts in the clinical area in which students are studying.

GUIDELINES FOR USING MULTIMEDIA

With the wealth of multimedia available for clinical teaching, the teacher should first evaluate the quality and appropriateness of the multimedia for the intended learning outcomes. Not all multimedia are of high quality nor are they appropriate for the objectives or meeting learner needs. Other guidelines for using multimedia for clinical teaching are:

- Prepare objectives to be achieved through completion of the multimedia.
- Consider assigning or recommending selected parts of a multimedia program that are most appropriate for the learning outcomes rather than the entire program.
- When parts of a multimedia program are used and when students complete multiple learning activities, provide written guidelines for them to follow that include the sequence for completing the activities. These guidelines direct students through varied activities and segments of a program, similar to a map.
- Plan for some of the activities involving multimedia to be completed in pairs or small groups. Small group discussions about the content and possible answers to questions posed in the multimedia and the exchange of ideas about problems, approaches, and multiple ways of viewing clinical situations encourage problem solving, decision making, and critical thinking.
- Consider carefully the number of resources, hardware and software, needed for effective implementation of the multmedia. Programs completed in pairs and small groups often ease the burden for adequate hardware and software for the total number of students within the time limitations.
- Develop questions for students to answer as they progress through the multimedia and at the end of the instruction, with answers, if feedback questions and a posttest are not already included. Review the multimedia first, for many will have questions integrated throughout for student response. Questions also may be written to link the multimedia to the specific clinical objectives and help students relate the content to the clinical setting and types of clients for whom they are caring.
- Provide an opportunity for students to evaluate the multimedia in terms of quality, from a learner's perspective, and usefulness in developing knowledge and skills for clinical practice.

Modules

Self-paced modules are another means of individualizing the clinical instruction and providing for self-directed learning. Modules are self-contained units of instruction that are completed independently by the learner (Reilly & Oermann, 1992). Students progress through the module at their own rates of learning. They may omit certain parts of the module or learning activities in it, or they may repeat those parts until the content is mastered. Other advantages of modules are accessibility, portability, and self-responsibility for learning (Herrick, Jenkins, & Carlson, 1998).

Modules generally include a variety of multimedia, although they might also be developed in print form only. Typically, though, different media are incorporated in them. Modules begin by stating the purpose of the module and clinical objectives to be met by its completion. Modules usually include a pretest to determine which objectives have already been met and the most appropriate point in the module to begin the instruction. Components of self-paced modules are listed in Table 8.3.

For clinical practice, modules may be used by students to acquire essential knowledge for care of patients, to review content or skills associated with a clinical experience, and to meet individual learning needs. Modules are used increasingly in staff development for orientation and continuing education of staff (Bryant, 1997; Herrick et al., 1998). Schlomer, Anderson, and Shaw (1997) found no significant differences in posttest scores between nurses who completed a module and those who had a lecture on the same content.

Independent Study

Independent study allows the student freedom in deciding his or her own learning goals, strategies for learning, and how the learning outcomes will be evaluated as part of the clinical course. The teacher and student typically collaborate on the objectives to be met through independent study so they relate to the clinical goals and are reasonable within the time frame. A contract may be established between the teacher and the student outlining the goals to be met through the independent study project, types of learning activities to be completed, evaluation methods and products of learning to be submitted as part of the clinical course, and dates for completion of these. Independent study is particularly useful when students want to explore a new area of clinical practice or a patient problem and interventions in depth.

SUMMARY

Many clinical objectives and competencies may be met by the students themselves through self-directed learning activities. Whether planned by the teacher as part of the clinical activities or recommended to meet specific learning needs, self-directed activities are intended for completion by the students on their own. These activities are typically self-contained units

Table 8.3 Components of Self-Paced Modules

Purpose of module
Objectives of module and relationship to clinical practice
Pretest for determining objectives already met
Self-directed learning activities incorporating multimedia
Feedback questions with answers for students to monitor their progress
Posttest
Additional learning activities and resources for learning

that students complete independently, often in a setting of their choice and according to their own time frame. Self-directed activities encourage them to assume responsibility for their own learning, an important outcome of nursing programs.

Self-directed activities may be completed by all students to meet certain clinical objectives or by students on an individual basis to reflect their particular learning needs. Similar to other types of learning activities, they should be consistent with the clinical objectives.

In planning self-directed activities, the teacher should consider the resources needed for their implementation. These resources include costs for developing materials, purchasing commercially available materials, and supporting software and hardware; equipment needed; space such as a computer laboratory; other requirements associated with a particular technology; and resources needed by students, such as Internet access. The time required for completion is another consideration in planning these activities for a course.

Self-directed activities are categorized as instructional media, such as videotapes; multimedia, including computer-assisted instruction, interactive videodisc, CD-ROM, virtual reality, and the Internet; modules; and independent study. Instructional media and multimedia promote learning through different senses, making it easier to comprehend difficult concepts. Media and multimedia that depict patient care scenarios help students understand how concepts and theories are used in practice and give them an idea of what a clinical situation is like. This vicarious experience prepares learners for the reality of clinical practice.

Multimedia are the combination of video, audio, text, and graphics that are presented using computer technology. Multimedia for use in clinical teaching are developing rapidly; there are tremendous possibilities for self-directed activities on the World Wide Web to support clinical learning. It is up to the teacher to be creative and willing to integrate these new technologies into clinical courses.

REFERENCES

Adsit, K. I. (1996). Multimedia in nursing and patient education. *Orthopaedic Nursing, 15,* 59–63.

Billings, D. M. (1996). Distance education in nursing. *Computers in Nursing, 14,* 211–212, 217.

Bridges, A., & Thede, L. Q. (1996). Nursing education resources on the World Wide Web. *Nurse Educator, 21*(5), 11–15.

Bryant, G. A. (1997). Suggestions for a competency-based orientation for an orthopaedic unit. *Orthopaedic Nursing, 16,* 67–75.

Carlton, K. E. H. (1996). Implications for nursing education: A virtual Mrs. Chase and cyberspace learning. *Computers in Nursing, 14,* 148–149.

Carlton, K. H., Ryan, M. E., & Siktberg, L. L. (1998). Designing courses for the Internet. *Nurse Educator, 23*(3), 45–50.

Clark, C. E. (1998). Teaching and learning at a distance. In D. M. Billings & J. A. Halstead (Eds.), *Teaching in nursing* (pp. 331–346). Philadelphia: Saunders.

Davis, K. A. (1998). Development and evaluation of computer-based training for pre/post human immunodeficiency virus test counseling. *Journal of Nursing Staff Development, 14,* 69–72.

DeAmicis, P. A. (1997). Interactive videodisc instruction is an alternative method for learning and performing a critical nursing skill. *Computers in Nursing, 15,* 155–158.

Edwards, M. J. A. (1995). Using computers in basic nursing education, continuing education, and patient education. In M. J. Ball, K. J. Hannah, S. K. Newbold, & J. V. Douglas (Eds.), *Nursing informatics: Where caring and technology meet* (pp. 350–361). New York: Springer-Verlag.

Falk, D. R., & Carlson, H. L. (1995). *Multimedia in higher education.* Medford, NJ: Learning Information.

Gayeski, D. M. (Ed.). (1993). *Multimedia for learning.* Englewood Cliffs, NJ: Educational Technology Publications.

Gee, P. R., Peterson, G. M., Martin, J. L. S., & Reeve, J. F. (1998). Development and evaluation of a computer-assisted instruction package in clinical pharmacology for nursing students. *Computers in Nursing, 16,* 37–44.

Gillham, D. (1998). Using hypertext to facilitate nurse education. *Computers in Nursing, 16,* 95–98.

Hedberg, J., Brown, C., & Arrighi, M. (1997). Interactive multimedia and web-based learning: Similarities and differences. In B. H. Khan (Ed.), *Wed-based instruction* (pp. 47–58). Englewood Cliffs, NJ: Educational Technology Publications.

Herrick, C. A., Jenkins, T. B., & Carlson, J. H. (1998). Using self-directed learning modules. *Journal of Nursing Staff Development, 14*, 73–80.

Khan, B. H. (Ed.). (1997). *Wed-based instruction.* Englewood Cliffs, NJ: Educational Technology Publications.

Ludy, J. E. (1998). Software reviews: SimBioSys Pulmonary Function Test. *Computers in Nursing, 16*, 181–183.

McGonigle, D., & Mastrian, K. (1998). Learning along the way: Cyberspacial quests. *Nursing Outlook, 46*, 81–86.

Nitko, A. J. (1996). *Educational assessment of students* (2nd ed.). Englewood Cliffs, NJ: Prentice-Hall.

Oermann, M. H. (1990). Research on teaching methods. *Annual review of research in nursing education* (pp. 1–31). New York: National League for Nursing.

Oermann, M. H., & Gaberson, K. B. (1998). *Evaluation and testing in nursing education.* New York: Springer.

Reilly, D. E., & Oermann, M. H. (1992). *Clinical teaching in nursing education* (2nd ed.). New York: National League for Nursing.

Riley, J. B. (1996). Educational applications. In V. K. Saba & K. A. McCormick (Eds.), *Essentials of computers for nurses* (2nd ed., pp. 527–573). New York: McGraw-Hill.

Schlomer, R. S., Anderson, M. A., & Shaw, R. (1997). Teaching strategies and knowledge retention. *Journal of Nursing Staff Development, 13*, 249–253.

Shockley, J., & Graveley, E. (1998). IAVD Series for Nursing Leadership and Management. *Computers in Nursing, 16*, 75–77.

Strauss, S. (1995). Cybersickness: The side effects of virtual reality. *Technology Review, 98*, 14–16.

Thomson, M. (1998). Multimedia anatomy and physiology lectures for nursing students. *Computers in Nursing, 16*, 101–108.

Van Dusen, G. E. (1997). *The virtual campus: Technology and reform in higher education.* Washington, DC: George Washington University.

Yoder, M. E. (1994). Preferred learning style and educational technology: Linear vs. interactive video. *Nursing & Health Care, 15*, 128–132.

Zwirn, E. E. (1998). Media, multimedia, and computer-mediated learning. In D. M. Billings & J. A. Halstead (Eds.), *Teaching in nursing* (pp. 315–329). Philadelphia: Saunders.

9

Learning Laboratories

Learning laboratories are used for a variety of purposes in clinical nursing education. The learning laboratory may be called a learning resource center, a skills laboratory, a college or campus laboratory, an instructional laboratory, a competency laboratory, or a mock hospital (Corder, 1991; Hodson-Carlton, 1998; Infante, 1985). This chapter describes purposes and types of learning laboratories and suggests ways to use these resources effectively in clinical nursing education.

PURPOSES AND TYPES OF LEARNING LABORATORIES

A learning laboratory may have a single, limited purpose, such as skill practice before entering the clinical environment, or it may serve multiple functions as a learning resource center. The scope of functions varies among nursing education programs depending on institutional mission, curriculum structure, and available resources.

Skill Development and Practice

The traditional use of the learning laboratory is for skill development prior to application in the clinical area. Infante (1985) differentiated the college laboratory from the clinical laboratory. In the college laboratory, the student develops and practices psychomotor and intellectual skills in preparation for transfer to real clinical practice situations in the clinical laboratory. The college laboratory provides controlled conditions under which students can learn and assemble skill components, test various approaches to performing the skill, develop speed and accuracy in skill performance, and make errors without harm to patients. It is an ideal setting for discovery, problem-based, and trial-and-error learning strategies. Learning in the college laboratory does not take the place of clinical learning; each is used for a specific purpose (Infante, 1985).

Skill development starts with prerequisite knowledge acquired in classroom and independent learning activities. Then students learn to handle the equipment and practice parts of the skill. Performance at this stage usually is slow and awkward; students may perform steps out of sequence, stop frequently to ask questions, and violate underlying principles such as asepsis. With repeated practice, however, performance becomes more accurate and coordinated. It usually is at this point that students are ready to enter the clinical area and to learn how to adapt the skill to meet the needs of particular patients. For example, the student practices the skill of intramuscular injection first in the skills laboratory. The student learns to select the proper size syringe and needle, withdraw the appropriate amount of medication into the syringe, select and clean the injection site on a mannequin, and administer the medication. The student may omit steps, contaminate sterile equipment, and select an inappropriate injection site, all without harm. When the student has learned all components of the skill and is able to assemble them into a smooth, coordinated performance, the next step is to enter the clinical area and learn how to adapt the skill to administer an intramuscular injection to a young child or an emaciated adult.

The skill practice laboratory also provides opportunities for formative evaluation of skill performance with plentiful feedback to the learner. Learner performance may be observed by a laboratory assistant or teacher, or the performance can be audiotaped or videotaped for later critique by the learner, the teacher, or both. For example, a student may audiotape a practice interview of a peer to obtain a health history. The audiotape may be reviewed by the student alone, who self-evaluates the performance and decides whether another practice interview is needed and if so, which interviewing skills need to be improved and how. The next audiotaped interview may be shared with the teacher for critique. The student would use the teacher's feedback as well as self-evaluation to determine if further practice is needed.

Because a skills laboratory allows students to learn and practice new skills in an environment where mistakes produce no harmful effects, student anxiety related to skill performance often is reduced (Hanson, 1993). Reilly and Oermann (1992) described skill learning as an egocentric process. The learner needs to have a sense of self as coordinated and in control before demonstrating a new skill in public. Excessive anxiety about performance evaluation also can interfere with learning; learners often ask questions of their peers rather than risk being judged as unprepared by their teachers (Packer, 1994). Anxiety can be reduced by providing opportunities for learners to practice the skill in relative privacy without the distractions of the actual clinical setting, to make mistakes without fear of embarrassment, and to repeat the skill as many times as necessary to feel confident. In the learning laboratory, teachers can use humor, mental imagery, and other strategies to reduce anxiety and improve self-confidence (Bucher, 1993; Doheny, 1993; Robbins, 1994).

Thus, use of a skill practice laboratory increases the effectiveness and efficiency of later clinical activities, produces more knowledgeable and skilled performance in the clinical area, allows the teacher's time to be used effectively, and reduces student anxiety about skill performance (Infante, 1985).

Multipurpose Learning Resource Center

In addition to serving as a skills practice laboratory, the learning resource center (LRC) provides resources for independent or guided development of intellectual skills, individual or group use of instructional media, and preparation for licensure or certification. The modern LRC is a multifunctional teaching and learning center for students of all levels (Hodson-Carlton, 1998).

LRCs may provide resources such as instructional media (audio- and videotape recorders and players, projectors, video- and audiotape collections), patient teaching materials, reference books and journals, photocopy equipment, computer hardware and software for computer-assisted instruction and simulations, and models for student and teacher use.

Thus, an LRC allows students to develop knowledge and skill necessary for theory-based practice and serves as the bridge between the science and the practice of nursing (Hanson, 1993). Students can develop and integrate a number of skills and practice them in a safe environment, with or without the teacher's guidance (Corder, 1991). An LRC offers facilities for teaching and learning in the cognitive, psychomotor, and affective domains (Morton, 1997).

USING LEARNING LABORATORIES EFFECTIVELY

Learning laboratories are best used in combination with classroom, independent learning, and clinical activities to produce desired outcomes. The following example illustrates how activities in the LRC and clinical learning activities can be sequenced to allow students to achieve a learning objective:

Objective: Carries out nursing interventions to assess and relieve respiratory distress.

Learning resource center activities	Clinical activities
Listen to audiotapes of normal and abnormal lung sounds.	Practice physical assessment of the chest and upper airway on selected patients of various ages.
View videotape of physical assessment of chest and upper airway.	Assess three patients with respiratory distress due to acute or chronic pulmonary disease.
Practice physical assessment of chest and upper airway on peers.	Formulate nursing diagnoses related to respiratory distress.
Practice physical assessment of simulated patient with respiratory distress.	Intervene to position patients and provide oxygen therapy.
Manipulate oxygen delivery equipment; apply oxygen mask to mannequin.	Compare assessment findings and patient outcomes at postclinical conference.
Practice positioning a simulated patient to relieve dyspnea.	

Skill Demonstration

A common use of learning laboratories is for psychomotor skill demonstration and return demonstration. Skill demonstrations are more effective in the learning laboratory than in the clinical area because the environment can be controlled, more learners can be accommodated, and the skill demonstration or any part of it can be repeated as many times as needed. Necessary materials can be assembled, stored, and reused for subsequent demonstrations and return demonstrations.

When demonstrating psychomotor skills to students, teachers should keep in mind that skilled performance has cognitive, motor, and affective components. It is important to recognize that cognitive intellectual processes are necessary for skill development; the learner must correctly perceive and interpret stimuli from the environment and choose and control the appropriate motor responses. Knowledge of results is essential if skill development is to occur. Therefore, the teacher should not only demonstrate the skill but allow learners to return the demonstration. The combination of oral feedback from the teacher and proprioceptive, visual, and tactile cues from the performance itself facilitates skill learning (Reilly & Oermann, 1992).

The teacher can be physically present for the demonstration or the learners can view a recorded demonstration on videotape or videodisc. One advantage of live demonstration is that learners can change their views of the performance by moving to a different vantage point; a disadvantage is that the teacher is only available at certain times. If the demonstration is recorded, however, each learner can view the whole performance or any part of it at a convenient time and as many times as desired.

While performing a live demonstration, the teacher should consider the learner's point of view. For example, if the teacher faces the learner while performing the skill, the learner's view is the mirror image of the teacher's; the teacher's right side is the learner's left. Therefore, when the teacher augments the demonstration with verbal cues, such as "Pick up the right glove with your left hand," the learner sees the action reversed, and this can interfere with the cognitive processing of the instructions. Instead, the teacher may take a position in front of or beside the learner and facing the same direction; the learner sees the action from the teacher's point of view.

Teachers can use checklists to evaluate return skill demonstrations and determine if the student is ready to apply the skill in an actual clinical setting. Table 9.1 shows an example of a skill checklist that could be used for formative evaluation in the skill practice laboratory. Note the criteria for successful performance that must be met before the student is permitted to enter the clinical area. A skill checklist also may be used as a reference tool during demonstration and practice of the skill and for self-evaluation (Hodson-Carlton, 1998).

Simulated Patients

Teachers often use a skills laboratory to provide simulations for students. Chapter 10 describes the use of written active case studies, computer simulations, and patient simulator software to teach cognitive and interpersonal skills.

A learning resource center also may provide live simulated patients for practice of psychomotor and interpersonal skills. Although it is common to practice new skills initially on peers, a simulated patient (SP) is a person who has been trained to feign symptoms and physical features of an actual patient realistically. A well-trained and experienced SP is proficient at discussing symptoms and history, portraying emotions, and exhibiting physical manifestations of illness such as aphasia, altered gait, or muscle

Table 9.1 Skill Performance Checklist

Surgical Scrub Skill Checklist

Performance criteria:

Follows steps in order

Keeps hands above the level of elbows at all times

Avoids wetting scrub clothing (bends forward at waist, holds elbows over sink)

Does not touch any part of sink once scrub has begun

Identifies and corrects breaks in technique

Procedure steps:

- Rolls up sleeves, tucks top into pants
- Removes watch, rings
- Obtains and opens scrub brush
- Turns water on
- Wets hands and arms
- Lathers fingernails with soap from sponge
- Cleans cuticles and under fingernails with cuticle stick
- Discards cuticle stick
- 20 horizontal strokes to fingernails; both hands
- 10 vertical strokes to each of 4 surfaces of each finger; both hands
- 10 circular strokes to palm; both hands
- 10 circular strokes to back of hand; both hands
- 10 vertical strokes to each of 4 surfaces of each forearm; both arms
- 10 vertical strokes to upper arm, 2 inches above elbow; both arms
- 10 horizontal strokes to elbow; both arms
- Discards brush
- Rinses each hand and arm thoroughly, fingertips to elbow

weakness, thereby offering students realistic learning opportunities without risk of harm to actual patients. SPs also may simulate family members of patients, allowing students to practice interactions such as teaching and interviewing. The student may practice psychomotor skills such as a pelvic examination, trying different approaches to organizing the steps of the procedure, and providing comfort for the patient. The SP also gives positive and negative feedback to the student from the patient's perspective, articulating how the patient felt and how the student's behavior affected those feelings. The student's interaction with the SP also can be audiotaped or videotaped for later review by the student, instructor, or both.

One advantage to using SPs is repeatability; the patient can be examined many times by the same or different students, with the same signs and symptoms displayed. Another advantage is controllability. The complexity, intensity, and timing of the situation can be chosen to fit the needs and abilities of the student. SPs can be paid professional actors or volunteers such as elderly adults from a senior center in the community served by the school. Health professionals usually do not make good SPs because their enactment of the patient role tends to be influenced by their own experience. The clinical teacher usually is responsible for selecting, training, and evaluating the SPs.

Scheduling Learning Laboratory Activities

Learning laboratories should be open during a wide range of hours, including evenings and weekends. Students should be able to schedule practice times when their academic, work, and personal schedules permit. Clinical teachers for each course might designate a minimum number of hours to be spent in college lab activities, but students should feel free to add hours according to their individual needs. The proportion of learning laboratory hours to clinical practice hours should change from beginning to end of the educational program. Planned and optional learning laboratory activities typically involve more time than clinical activities at the beginning of the program. At the end of the program, when students are spending most of their time in integrative clinical activities, they may need to spend little or no time in the skill practice laboratory (Reilly & Oermann, 1992).

RESOURCE REQUIREMENTS

Clinical teachers often are involved in planning and equipping a learning laboratory to meet the needs of learners and instructors. Resource needs for learning laboratories depend on their purpose and function, but in general, all learning laboratories require physical space, equipment, personnel, and financial resources.

Physical Space and Equipment

The amount of space required depends on whether the laboratory will be used only for skills practice or for multipurpose functions. Physical space should include at least a room that simulates a health care setting, for practice of psychomotor skills, and a separate space for use of audiovisual media. A skills practice area should simulate the current reality of health care. Thus, if students are to be prepared to function competently in clinical areas such as acute care, critical care, extended care, home care, and community settings, the practice laboratory should contain equipment and supplies that would be common to those settings (Hodson-Carlton, 1998). For example, if learners are to be prepared for practice in critical care units, the skills practice laboratory might contain a critical care bed, wall suction and oxygen outlets and equipment, a cardiac monitor, an infusion pump, a pulse oximeter, a ventilator, chest tube equipment, an electrocardiogram machine, rewarming equipment, cardiopulmonary resuscitation equipment, and mannequins that simulate cardiac arrhythmias (Morton, 1997). A practice area for skills used in a home care environment might include a table and chairs, a couch, and typical bedroom furniture.

If the laboratory is a multipurpose LRC, it usually requires additional space for computer hardware and software, a print resource library, storage of patient teaching materials, and the like.

Personnel

Almost every learning laboratory needs personnel to staff it at least part time. Clinical teachers should be available to students during scheduled hours to reinforce teaching, answer questions, and determine students' readiness for clinical activities. Additional teaching staff may be needed to prepare simulations, guide learning activities, answer questions, and provide feedback to learners when clinical teachers are not present. These additional support staff members could be graduate teaching assistants, part-time laboratory assistants, volunteer graduates of the school, and the like.

Other personnel whose services may be needed, depending on the purpose of the learning laboratory, include librarians, computer support staff, and audiovisual media specialists. Most LRCs require at least one faculty or staff position designated as LRC director, manager, supervisor, or coordinator. Depending on academic preparation and clinical and teaching experience, the LRC director may contribute to curriculum development and program evaluation related to the learning laboratory, teaching and evaluating psychomotor skills, planning for ongoing technological improvements, managing the physical facilities, supervising other support staff, grant writing, and conducting research (Hodson-Carlton, 1998).

Budget

The size and scope of learning laboratory activities also affect the required budget. The primary source for funding the learning laboratory usually is the supporting institution; however, grant funding is available from some sources for improving nursing education programs through development and improvement of learning resources

In addition to the usual overhead costs for lighting, heat, phone and computer lines, and the like, the budget must include funds for purchase, replacement, and maintenance of equipment; purchase of supplies; purchase of instructional media; and laundry, cleaning, and other maintenance costs. Salary costs for personnel, including the LRC director and laboratory teaching and support staff, must also be included. If trained simulated patients are hired, their fees and expenses are another item in the budget.

Partnerships may be developed in order to share costs of operating the learning laboratory. Some learning laboratories serve as interdisciplinary learning resource centers; students from a variety of health care disciplines such as medicine, physical therapy, and nursing may share practice space and equipment while they learn collaboratively (Hodson-Carlton, 1998). In addition to the cost-sharing benefit, such partnerships promote interdisciplinary education that prepares learners for the reality of practice in today's health care system.

SUMMARY

The learning laboratory, also called a learning resource center, a skills laboratory, a college or campus laboratory, an instructional laboratory, or a competency laboratory, serves a variety of purposes in clinical nursing education depending on the institutional mission, curriculum structure, and resources. A learning laboratory may have a limited purpose, such as skill practice before entering the clinical environment, or it may serve multiple functions as a learning resource center

The traditional use of the learning laboratory is for skill development. In the skills laboratory, the student develops and practices psychomotor and intellectual skills in preparation for transfer to real clinical practice situations. In the controlled conditions of the skills laboratory, students can learn and assemble skill components, test various approaches to performing the skill, develop speed and accuracy, and make errors without harm to patients. The skill practice laboratory also provides opportunities for formative evaluation of skill performance with feedback to the learner. Use of a skill practice laboratory also reduces student anxiety about skill performance. In addition to serving as a skills practice laboratory, the learning resource center may provide resources such as instructional media, patient teaching materials, print resources, computer hardware and software, and models for student and teacher use.

Learning laboratories commonly are used for psychomotor skill demonstration and return demonstration. Skill demonstrations are more effective in the learning laboratory than in the clinical area because the environment can be controlled, more learners can be accommodated, and the skill demonstration or any part of it can be repeated as many times as needed. Demonstrations may be live or recorded. With a live demonstration, learners can change their views of the performance. If the demonstration is recorded, each learner can view the performance at a convenient time and repeat it as desired. While performing live demonstrations, teachers should position themselves so that the learners' view is consistent with the teachers' verbal directions. Skill checklists can be used as guidelines for practice and evaluation tools.

Simulated patients who have been trained to feign symptoms and physical features of actual patients may be provided for practice of psychomotor and interpersonal skills. A well-trained simulated patient can discuss symptoms and history, portray emotions, and exhibit physical manifestations of illness, thereby offering students realistic, risk-free learning opportunities.

Learning laboratories should be open during a wide range of hours to meet students' individual needs. The proportion of learning laboratory hours to clinical practice hours should change from the beginning to the end of the educational program; more time is spent in the learning laboratory at the beginning of a program, and more time is spent in clinical activities at the end.

Clinical teachers often are involved in planning and equipping a learning laboratory. Resource needs depend on the purpose and function of the learning laboratory. All learning laboratories require physical space, equipment, personnel, and financial resources. A skills practice area should simulate the current reality of health care, with equipment and supplies consistent with those likely to be found in the setting in which learners will practice. Personnel include teaching and support staff; many multipurpose learning centers require a director whose responsibilities may include grant writing and learning center development. Multidisciplinary learning centers allow for cost-sharing while preparing learners to function collaboratively in today's health care systems.

REFERENCES

Bucher, L. (1993). The effects of imagery abilities and mental rehearsal on learning a nursing skill. *Journal of Nursing Education, 32*, 318–324.

Corder, J. B. (1991). Campus clinical: An alternative clinical activity. *Journal of Nursing Education, 30*, 420–421.

Doheny, M. O. (1993). Mental practice: An alternative approach to teaching motor skills. *Journal of Nursing Education, 32*, 260–264.

Hanson, G. F. (1993). Refocusing the skills laboratory. *Nurse Educator, 18*(2), 10–12.

Hodson-Carlton, K. E. (1998). The learning resource center. In D. M. Billings & J. A. Halstead (Eds.), *Teaching in nursing: A guide for faculty* (pp. 301–314). Philadelphia: Saunders.

Infante, M. S. (1985). *The clinical laboratory in nursing education* (2nd ed.). New York: Wiley.

Morton, P. G. (1997). Using a critical care simulation laboratory to teach students. *Critical Care Nurse, 17*(6), 66–69.

Packer, J. L. (1994). Education for clinical practice: An alternative approach. *Journal of Nursing Education, 33,* 411–416.

Reilly, D. E., & Oermann, M. H. (1992). *Clinical teaching in nursing education* (2nd ed.). New York: National League for Nursing.

Robbins, L. (1994). Using humor to enhance learning in the skills laboratory. *Nurse Educator, 19*(3), 39–42.

Stokes, L. (1998). Teaching in the clinical setting. In D. M. Billings & J. A. Halstead (Eds.), *Teaching in nursing: A guide for faculty* (pp. 281–297). Philadelphia: Saunders.

10

Simulations and Games for Clinical Learning

Simulations create realistic situations for students to meet the outcomes of clinical practice and develop essential skills without the demands of caring for an actual patient. As clinical practice has become more complex, simulations provide a means of gaining practice experience without having to contend with the realities of a clinical situation. Other experiential methods such as role play and games serve similar purposes, providing learning activities for students to develop cognitive and interpersonal skills and gain new knowledge useful for clinical practice. Games also add variety to the learning activities, particularly for postconferences when students may be fatigued from their clinical activities and may have difficulty discussing complex concepts.

This chapter describes three experiential methods for clinical teaching: simulations, role play, and games. These methods may be used as planned activities to learn new concepts and skills as part of clinical practice or as supplemental activities for review and practice.

SIMULATIONS

A simulation creates a scenario that mimics a real-life situation. For this reason, simulations provide a way for students to gain experience in problem solving and decision making without the realities and demands of an actual clinical situation. There are many clinical situations for which expert knowledge and skills are needed, such as life-threatening events.

Simulations allow the student to gain experience in thinking through these situations and acting out the nurse's role.

Another important use of simulations is for practice of psychomotor, interpersonal, and other skills. With simulations students can learn how to use equipment, perform a procedure, and carry out complex technological skills in a laboratory environment rather than with actual patients. Simulations may be used for initial learning of the skill, for continued practice to refine the skill further, and for reinforcement and review at a later time. For procedures involving equipment and supplies, simulations are cost-effective if the supplies can be reused by the learner and by other students. For interpersonal and leadership skills, simulations provide essential experience for developing these abilities and for student self-evaluation.

Hanna (1991) also suggested that simulations are valuable for affective learning. Simulations may be developed for students to experience conflicting situations requiring an assessment of their own values. Through a simulation students may examine their feelings, beliefs, and values before encountering a similar situation in their own clinical practice. Simulations may be used for learners to develop an awareness of what a situation would be like for a patient, family, and staff; these simulations are most appropriate for affective learning and value development.

With a simulation the teacher can control the clinical situation more easily than in actual practice and, as a result, can adapt the learning activity to individual student needs. Students who need extra practice, for instance with psychomotor skills, can repeat performance until mastery is achieved. This is an important outcome of using simulations because many times students do not have sufficient experiences in clinical practice to refine their skills further. Skill learning opportunities either are not available or students need more practice. When using simulations for development of skills, the teacher can provide immediate feedback, can guide students in performing the skill accurately, and can reinforce their learning. Often in the clinical setting, the teacher is not available for immediate feedback and reinforcement.

Prior to beginning a simulation, students need clear expectations as to the learning outcomes and how they relate to the clinical objectives. These outcomes keep the simulation focused, preventing a drift away from the intended goals of the activity. When psychomotor skill learning is involved, students should have at the outset the performance criteria to be met. With every simulation, students should have guidelines as to how to progress through the simulated activities.

At the end of the simulation, a debriefing session or discussion should be held to

- emphasize the major learning outcomes from the simulated experience,
- reinforce learning that has occurred and relate it to the objectives,
- relate the simulation to actual clinical practice,
- identify where further learning is needed,
- discuss feelings generated through the simulation, and
- examine changes that may be needed in own behaviors to better meet patient needs.

The debriefing may be done on a one-to-one basis with the student or as a clinical group, depending on how the simulation was designed. For simulations completed by students individually in a learning laboratory, the teacher should include strategies, such as review questions, for students to assess their own achievement of the outcomes of the simulation and how their learning would be used in an actual clinical situation. For this latter purpose, short clinical scenarios for analysis provide an effective means of helping students relate their simulated experience to clinical practice.

Types of Simulations

There are different types of simulations appropriate for clinical learning activities and different combinations of these that are possible: active case studies, presented in paper-and-pencil format, as computer simulations, and using multimedia; models; and simulated patients using actors and other people to act out the role of a patient. Each of these types of simulations creates an experience that represents a real-life situation.

ACTIVE CASE STUDY

In the active case study method, information about a clinical situation is presented for analysis. The case may depict a situation for problem solving, decision making, or critical thinking, or it may require application of the concepts and theories being learned in class for its analysis. Information is gradually added to the case, asking for different types of decisions and further thinking for resolution of problems. Simulations using case studies may incorporate different scenarios that show how patient conditions and clinical situations change over time. In this way the case study more clearly reflects the reality of clinical practice. Through their analysis of the case study, students gain experience in thinking through these clinical scenarios and learn to solve hypothetical problems.

Glendon and Ulrich (1997) referred to active case studies as "unfolding cases." Unfolding cases present a scenario that changes, developing the case further. In this model, the unfolding case begins with a paragraph that sets the stage for the scenario. It includes background information about the client and focused questions. Students working in groups answer the questions, then share their responses with the other students. A second paragraph is then revealed that changes the scenario in some way. Students once again answer the related questions. This process continues, thereby developing the case into a simulation. The final step is a writing exercise in which students share individual reactions and reflect on the learning experience (Glendon & Ulrich, 1997). At this point the teacher can help students relate the simulated case to clinical practice.

Active case studies may be presented in paper-and-pencil format (see Table 10.1), as computer simulations, and using multimedia. Computer simulations have an added advantage in that feedback may be given on the consequences of the decisions made (Reilly & Oermann, 1992). In a computer simulation, students may be asked questions about the data presented in the case and required to select interventions; students then receive immediate feedback on their analysis and appropriateness of the chosen interventions. With some computer simulations, the patient's status and clinical situation are altered by the student's responses, thereby changing the scenario. This communicates to learners the results of their problem solving and decision making.

Patient simulator software provides realistic patients for students to analyze clinical and laboratory data, select interventions, and see the results of their treatments. Durbin (1998) reviewed patient simulator software, available on CD-ROM or diskettes, of a normal patient and 10 ill patients for diagnosis and treatment. The simulated patient comes to life when the program begins or a case is selected by the student. A "clinical view" window is included to represent a physiological monitoring screen in a critical care unit. Menus allow for performance of electrocardigrams (ECGs), physical examinations, and vital sign measurement; recording of relevant data; and selection of treatments. The mechanical ventilator offers seven ventilatory modes; the student controls the ventilator settings during the simulation. The simulator responds to the interventions selected by students so they can see the results of their treatments (Durbin, 1998).

Another type of patient simulator is designed to simulate critically ill patients and provide practice in evaluating and treating them. In this simulation students are presented with 12 critically ill patients. Each case includes a brief description of the patient, present illness, and past medical history. Students begin by reviewing the history and reading the bedside monitor display of ECG waveforms, pressure waveforms, and other data. There are multiple decisions possible as to treatment options, and flow sheets are automatically completed (Short, 1998).

Active case studies using multimedia such as interactive videodisc instruction (IVDI), as described in Chapter 8, present the clinical situation

Table 10.1 Simulation: Active Case Study

Example 1

Ms. D, 61 years old, is seen in the clinic with increasing shortness of breath. She has had three "chest colds" this month alone. You hear crackles in the lower bases of her lungs and expiratory wheezes.

1. What additional data would you collect in the initial assessment? Why are these data important?
2. What are Ms. D's priority problems? Name all likely problems.
3. How will the data you plan on collecting help you confirm them?

Three days later, Ms. D returns to the clinic with a high temperature, general weakness, and chills. Her white blood cell count is elevated. You notice that Ms. D is coughing more, and her sputum is a yellow-green color. She is admitted to the hospital with the diagnosis of pneumonia.

1. Describe nursing interventions for Ms. D and provide a rationale for them.
2. What outcomes will you measure to determine if Ms. D is progressing?

Ms. D improves and is told that she will be discharged. She begins to cry, telling the nurse, "I have no reason to go home. There is no one there to be with. Please don't make me go home." You remember from the medical record that Ms. D has a daughter who lives nearby. The daughter, however, did not visit her mother throughout the hospitalization.

1. How would you respond to Ms. D?
2. Describe three possible approaches you could take in response to Ms. D's concern about returning home. What are the consequences of each approach?
3. Which approach would you use? Why?

(continued)

Table 10.1 *(continued)*

Example 2

Mrs. P, 53 years old with a history of hypertension, was admitted to your unit after being found unconscious in her home by a neighbor. A computerized tomography (CT) scan indicated a subarachnoid hemorrhage. Arterial blood gases were pH 7.30, $PaCO_2$ 48 mm Hg, and PaO_2 58 mm Hg. Oxygen saturation was 71%. Mrs. P was intubated and placed on a ventilator. Ventilator settings were A/C 10, Vt 500, and FIO_2 50%. Your assessment shows right-sided motor weakness of 2/5 and left-sided motor strength of 5/5. Mrs. P is both agitated and confused. She has diffuse rales and pink sputum from the endotracheal tube.

1. Describe at least four different nursing interventions that should be included in Mrs. P's care.
2. Provide a rationale for each.
3. What action would you take *now*? Why?
4. Specify outcome criteria for evaluating the effectiveness of the intervention you selected.
5. What information presented in this situation is irrelevant to your decision making? Why?

Mrs. P becomes more agitated. What are possible causes of her agitation?

Later that day the physician orders a new drug for Mrs. P. You call the pharmacy to learn more about the drug and find that the amount ordered is more than twice the acceptable dose. The physician tells you to "give it anyway. The dose is okay for this patient."

1. What are different options for you at this time? Describe advantages and disadvantages of each.
2. How would you solve this dilemma?

Note. From M. H. Oermann (1998). How to assess critical thinking. *Dimensions of Critical Care Nursing, 17*(6), p. 6. Copyright 1998 by Springhouse. Adapted with permission.

(continued)

Table 10.1 *(continued)*

Example 3

C, who is 12 years old, lives in an urban area with his parents and three siblings. He was diagnosed with asthma 2 years ago. Skin tests confirmed allergies to a number of pollens, dust mites, and cats. His mother smokes one pack of cigarettes per day. C presents in the clinic with wheezing both at night and during the day. You hear audible wheezing as C speaks.

1. What questions will you ask and what data will you collect about C's wheezing?
2. Describe background information needed about C's health status.
3. What diagnostic tests should be ordered? Why?

Two weeks later C returns for a follow-up visit. He reports less wheezing. You listen to his lungs and hear a few end-expiratory wheezes at the bases, but overall C shows significant improvement. C is worried about becoming short of breath at school.

1. What are key areas to include in C's teaching plan?
2. How would you adapt your teaching methods considering C's age and developmental stage?
3. What strategies will you use in teaching C's mother about her smoking and its relationship to his asthma?

C progresses well until one day at school when he starts wheezing during recess. C is so short of breath, he has difficulty speaking.

1. What actions should the school nurse take *first*? Why?
2. What critical information about C's asthma should be in his medical records at school to guide the nurse in deciding on interventions? Why is this information important?
3. Develop an asthma management plan for C during school.

---

more realistically than does the paper-and-pencil format. With IVDI the student is able to view the client's progress in the simulated situation and "see" how the patient responds to different treatments and interventions. IVDI creates real-life simulations for students to identify data to be collected, analyze data, plan care, select interventions, and evaluate changes in client conditions, all with immediate feedback from the computer.

Simulations also may be developed with videotapes of patient scenarios for student analysis and to view a clinical situation prior to encountering it in practice. Or students may read cases, then act out roles and be videotaped on their performance. With all of these types of active case studies, students may carry out actual procedures and skills as part of the simulation.

MODELS

Another type of simulation involves the use of models, such as mannequins and models of the breast, for learning clinical skills and practicing procedures. Many models are available for developing clinical skills in nursing, such as cardiopulmonary resuscitation of adults and children, breast and testicular examinations, pelvic examination, and endotracheal intubation. These models allow students to practice their skills in a safe environment without distractions and to develop self-confidence in performing them.

SIMULATED PATIENTS

One other type of simulation uses actors, peers, or other people to portray the role of the patient. With this type, students may practice taking a health history, performing a physical examination, and other activities (Reilly & Oermann, 1992). Student performance may be videotaped for evaluation of skills by the faculty at a later time.

ROLE PLAY

Closely related to simulations is role play, in which the learner portrays a certain role as a way of experiencing that role or for developing communication and leadership skills. In role play the learner is directed as to the role to portray but usually is given freedom in acting it out. While students are portraying the assigned roles, other students in the clinical group observe and analyze the behaviors. For some objectives, students may be videotaped for self-assessment or for evaluation by the teacher.

Some guidelines for role play are:

- Develop the role play activity based on the objectives to be met.
- Describe the roles to be portrayed and the clinical situation, but keep this description brief so students have freedom to act out the roles.

- Limit the time to approximately 15 minutes to keep the role play focused on the objectives.
- Provide guidelines for the analysis of the role play for students who are observing it. These guidelines should help students focus their attention as they observe the role play.
- Discuss the role play, the behaviors observed, and how the role play reflects the learning outcomes. This debriefing is essential for students to relate the role play experience to the intended objectives.
- Avoid discussion of the students' acting ability and instead focus on the learning to be gained from the role play activity.

GAMES

A game is a contest with rules, goals, and activities to perform (Reilly & Oermann, 1992). While the theory of gaming was introduced many years ago, games have become more prevalent recently with the shift toward experiential learning strategies. Games may be played individually, such as crossword puzzles, or as a group, for instance, board games. Speers (1993) described how to develop crossword puzzles for teaching new terminology and definitions and for mandated education. Games also may be played as a group. Ingram, Ray, Landeen, and Keane (1998) described "Let's Hypothesize," a board game to increase students' abilities in hypothesis and issue generation during problem-based learning.

Games are effective for practice and review and are fun to play (Henry, 1997). They may increase motivation and interest in a topic and actively involve the learner, allowing the student to control the learning environment. Games add diversity to teaching and, as such, are particularly appropriate for content that is repetitive (Bradbury-Golas & Carson, 1994; Henry, 1997). They are effective strategies for use in postconference and during learning activities when students need change to keep motivated and interested. It is important, though, with any gaming strategy that students have the prerequisite knowledge and skills for completing the game and learning from it.

The debriefing session at the conclusion of the game provides the avenue for emphasizing key points learned in the game and how they relate to clinical practice. Questions to help the teacher plan games as clinical learning activities are found in Table 10.2.

Saethang and Kee (1998) described a gaming strategy that combined games and case studies for teaching the administration of drugs. In this method, nurses first read a case study related to the topic; the games follow this case study. Learners are divided into competing teams. A game board is used, with six different wedges representing drug dosage, action

Table 10.2 Planning for Games as Clinical Learning Activities

Consider these points:

- Does the game relate to the clinical objectives?
- Does the game assist students in developing clinical knowledge and competencies?
- Does it teach new content or provide a review of content already learned?
- Does the game assist students in developing decision-making and problem-solving skills?
- Do students have the prerequisite knowledge and skills for completing the game?
- Will students be motivated by the game format?
- Is the game interesting to play?
- Can the game be completed in the time frame allotted?
- Does the game require equipment, supplies, and props? Are these available? Reusable? Affordable?
- Is there physical space to play the game?
- What are the requirements of the game, such as number of participants, and are these appropriate for the learning situation?
- What is the preparation time for the teacher for planning the game? Setting up the game? Cleaning up?
- What are important questions for the debriefing?

of the drug, nursing implications, drug classification, side effects, and generic name. The game format includes questions about these categories of information, with points acquired for correct responses.

Many games are combined with simulation to allow students to experience a situation but in a game format. Hanna (1991) described a simulation game as a variation of simulation that adds the element of competition and the goal of winning. One example is Star Power, a simulation game in which people progress from one level of society to another by trading with others (Simulation Training Systems, 1998). Star Power is an effective simulation game for helping students understand the proper uses of power. Another simulation game, BaFa' BaFa', is geared toward developing affective outcomes related to cultural awareness. In BaFa' BaFa', students are sensitized to cultural diversity and learn what it feels like to be "different."

SUMMARY

Simulations create realistic scenarios for students to meet the outcomes of clinical practice and develop essential skills without the risks and demands of actual patient care. They provide a means of gaining practice experience without having to contend with the realities of a clinical situation. Other experiential methods such as role play and games serve similar purposes.

There are different types of simulations appropriate for clinical learning activities and different combinations of these that are possible: active case studies, presented in paper-and-pencil format, as computer simulations, and using multimedia; models; and simulated patients using actors and other people to act out the role of a patient. Each of these types of simulations creates a scenario that represents a real-life situation. Closely related to simulations is role play, in which the learner portrays a certain role as a way of experiencing that role or for developing communication and leadership skills.

Games are effective for practice and review and are fun to play. They actively involve the learner, allowing the student to control the learning environment. Games add diversity to teaching and, as such, are particularly appropriate for content that is repetitive. Many games are combined with simulation to allow students to experience a situation but in a game format. With all of these experiential learning activities, the debriefing session that follows the simulation, role play, or game is critical to discuss the learning outcomes and how these relate to the clinical objectives. In the debriefing students also examine how this new learning may be used in their own clinical practice.

REFERENCES

Bradbury-Golas, K., & Carson, L. (1994). Nursing skills fair: Gaining knowledge with fun and games. *Journal of Continuing Education in Nursing, 25,* 32–34.

Durbin, C. G. (1998). Patient simulator. *Journal of the American Medical Association, 279,* 1125.

Glendon, K., & Ulrich, D. L. (1997). Unfolding cases: An experiential learning model. *Nurse Educator, 22*(4), 15–18.

Hanna, D. R. (1991). Using simulations to teach clinical nursing. *Nurse Educator, 16*(2), 28–31.

Henry, J. M. (1997). Gaming: A teaching strategy to enhance adult learning. *Journal of Continuing Education in Nursing, 28,* 231–234.

Ingram, C., Ray, K., Landeen, J., & Keane, D. R. (1998). Evaluation of an educational game for health science students. *Journal of Nursing Education, 37,* 240–246.

Reilly, D. E., & Oermann, M. H. (1992). *Clinical teaching in nursing education.* New York: National League for Nursing.

Saethang, T., & Kee, C. C. (1998). A gaming strategy for teaching the use of critical cardiovascular drugs. *Journal of Continuing Education in Nursing, 29*, 61–65.

Short, B. (1998). Sim*BioSys* Clinics. [On-line.] Available: http://www.wwnurse.com/software_reviews/simbiosys_clinics.shtml

Simulation Training Systems. (1998). [On-line.] http://www.stsintl.com/edu_main.html

Speers, A. T. (1993). Crossword puzzles: A teaching strategy for critical care nursing. *Dimensions of Critical Care Nursing, 12*(6), 52–55.

11

Case Method, Case Study, and Grand Rounds

Clinical practice provides opportunities for students to gain the knowledge and skills needed to care for patients; develop values important in professional practice; and develop cognitive skills for processing and analyzing data, deciding on problems and interventions, and evaluating their effectiveness. Case method, case study, and grand rounds are effective means in developing these learning outcomes. Case method and case study describe a clinical situation, developed around an actual or hypothetical patient, for student review and critique. In case method the case provided for analysis is generally shorter and more specific than in case study. Case studies are more comprehensive in nature, thereby presenting a complete picture of the patient and clinical situation.

With each of these clinical teaching methods, students apply concepts and theories to practice situations, identify actual and potential problems, propose varied approaches for solving them, weigh different decisions possible, and arrive at judgments as to the effectiveness of interventions. As such, case method and study and grand rounds provide experience for students in thinking through different client situations. Students gain a perspective of patients, families, and communities for whom they may be responsible in future practice.

SKILL IN PROBLEM SOLVING

There are varied perspectives of problem solving, decision making, and critical thinking. In general, problem solving is the ability to solve clinical problems, some relating to the patient and others that arise from clinical practice. Problem solving begins with recognizing and defining the problem, gathering data to clarify it further, developing solutions, and evaluating their effectiveness (Oermann & Gaberson, 1998).

Viewed as a cognitive *skill*, problem solving can be developed through repeated experiences, with real patients, such as in grand rounds, or simulated cases, such as case method and study. The student does not need to provide hands-on care to develop problem-solving skills. Observing and discussing the patient during grand rounds and analyzing cases provide essential experience in problem solving. These methods give students a perspective of what to expect in an actual clinical situation, typical problems the client may experience, interventions that should be considered for care, and similarities and differences across clinical situations.

Complexity of Cases for Review

Cases for review and critique may be of varying levels of complexity. Some cases may be designed with the problems readily apparent. With these cases the problem is described clearly, and sufficient information is included to guide decisions on how to intervene. Nitko (1996) called these cases well structured, providing an opportunity for students to apply concepts to a patient situation and develop an understanding of how they are used in clinical practice. Cases of this type link knowledge presented in class and through readings to practice situations.

Most patient care situations, however, are not that easily solved. In clinical practice the problems are sometimes difficult to identify, or the nurse may be confident as to the patient's problem but unsure how to intervene. These are problems in Schön's (1990) swampy lowland, ones that do not lend themselves to resolution by a technical and rational approach. These are cases that vary from the way the problems and solutions were presented in class and through readings. For cases such as these, the principles learned in class may not readily apply, and critical thinking is required for analysis and resolution.

Nitko (1996) referred to these as ill-structured cases, describing problems that reflect real-life clinical situations faced by students. With ill-structured cases for review and critique, different problems may be possible, there may be an incomplete data set to determine the problem, or the problem may be clear but multiple solutions may be possible. Table 11.1 presents examples of a well-structured and an ill-structured case.

Table 11.1 Well-Structured and Ill-Structured Problems

Well-Structured Problem

Mrs. D, 53 years old, complains of bad headaches for the last month. The headaches occur about 2 times per week, usually in the late morning. Initially the pain began as a throbbing at her right temple. Her headaches now affect either her right or left eye and temple. The pain is so severe, she usually "goes to bed." Mrs. D complains of her neck hurting, and the nurse notes tenderness in the posterior neck.

1. What type(s) of headache might Mrs. D be experiencing?
2. Describe additional data that should be collected from Mrs. D.
3. Select one intervention that might be used for Mrs. D. Provide evidence for its use.

Ill-Structured Problem

Ms. J, 35 years old, calls for an appointment because she fell yesterday at home. She has a few bruises from her fall and a "tingling feeling in her legs." Ms. J had been at the eye doctor's last week for double vision.

1. What additional data should be collected from Ms. J? Why are these data important?
2. List laboratory and diagnostic tests for Ms. J. Why should these be ordered?
3. What are possible diagnoses for Ms. J to be considered?

SKILL IN DECISION MAKING

Case method and study and grand rounds also assist students in developing decision-making skills. Decision making involves considering different alternatives, weighing the consequences of each, then arriving at a decision or choice as to the best alternative for the situation. With case method and study, clinical situations may be described that require a decision. Questions that accompany the case ask students to consider the alternatives possible and consequences of each, then arrive at a decision following this analysis.

SKILL IN CRITICAL THINKING

Critical thinking enables the nurse to make reasoned and informed judgments in the practice setting and decide what to do in a given situation (Facione & Facione, 1996). It is reflective thinking about patient problems without one solution (Kataoka-Yahiro & Saylor, 1994; Whiteside, 1997). Through critical thinking the learner

- considers multiple perspectives to care,
- critiques different approaches possible in a clinical situation,
- arrives at judgments after considering multiple possibilities,
- raises questions about issues to clarify them further, and
- resolves issues with a well thought out approach (Oermann, 1997, 1998; Oermann & Gaberson, 1998).

Another perspective of critical thinking involves its use in problem solving and decision making. Through critical thinking, students differentiate relevant from irrelevant data, identify cues in data and cluster them, propose varied diagnoses that might be possible, and decide on additional data needed for determining the diagnosis. In terms of interventions, critical thinking enables them to compare different approaches to care, weigh alternatives, and decide on the best approach considering these possibilities. The ability to think critically and reason logically underlies effective clinical practice (Sedlak, 1997).

CASE METHOD

Case method and case study serve similar purposes in clinical teaching—they provide a simulated case for student review and critique. In case method the case provided for analysis is generally shorter and more specific than in case study.

Cases may be developed around actual or hypothetical patients. Depending on how the case is written, case method is effective for applying concepts and theories to clinical practice and for promoting problem solving, decision making, and critical thinking. Case method is a useful strategy for helping students learn how to analyze a case, identify problems and solutions, compare alternate decisions, and arrive at conclusions about different aspects of patient care (Oermann & Gaberson, 1998). Examples of case method are presented in Table 11.2.

Table 11.2 Examples of Case Method

Problem Solving

Mrs. F has moderate dementia. She lets the nurse practitioner (NP) do a pelvic examination because she has a "woman's problem." The examination shows an anterior wall prolapse. After helping Mrs. F get dressed, the NP finds that Mrs. F has stress incontinence. Urine begins leaking to the floor, and Mrs. F appears embarrassed.

1. List and prioritize Mrs. F's problems. Provide a rationale for how the problems are prioritized.
2. Develop a plan of care for Mrs. F.

A 40-year-old woman with diabetes was admitted with a subarachnoid hemorrhage. A middle cerebral artery aneurysm was clipped without complications 3 days after her symptoms began. The patient was recovering until she developed right-sided weakness and aphasia. Her temperature is now 39°C, pulse 100, respirations 18, and blood pressure 190/100. Cranial computed tomography (CT) scan showed stable cerebral blood flow, no rebleeding, and flow deficit in left middle cerebral artery distribution.

1. What is the primary cause of the neurologic deficit? Provide an explanation for your answer.
2. What are options in treatment?
3. Describe nursing interventions for this patient.

Note. From *Critical Care Pearls* (2nd ed., p. 19), by S. A. Sahn and J. E. Heffner, 1998, Philadelphia: Hanley & Belfus. Copyright 1998 by Hanley & Belfus. Adapted with permission.

You are working in a pediatrician's office. Mrs. C brings her son in for a checkup after a severe asthma attack a month ago that required emergency care. When you ask Mrs. C how her son is doing, she begins to cry softly. She tells you she is worried about his having another asthma attack and this time not recovering from it. When the pediatrician enters the examination room, Mrs. C is still crying. The physician says, "What's wrong? Look at him. He's doing great."

1. What would you say to Mrs. C, if anything, in this situation?
2. What would you say to the pediatrician, if anything?

(continued)

Table 11.2 *(continued)*

You have a new patient, 81 years old, with congestive heart failure. The referral to your home health agency indicates that Mr. A has difficulty breathing, tires easily, and has edema in both legs, making it difficult for him to get around. He lives alone.

1. What are the patient problems you anticipate for Mr. A? Include a rationale for each of these problems.

At your first home visit, you find Mr. A sitting in a chair with his feet on the floor. During your assessment, he gets short of breath talking with you and has to stop periodically to "catch his breath."

1. Describe at least three different nursing interventions that could be used in Mr. A's care. Provide a rationale for each.

2. Specify outcome criteria for evaluating the effectiveness of the interventions you selected.

3. What would you teach Mr. A?

4. Identify one research study that relates to Mr. A's care. Critique the study and describe whether or not you could use the findings in caring for Mr. A and similar patients.

Decision Making

Mrs. M is a 42-year-old elementary school teacher with a history of inflammatory bowel disease. She calls the clinic for an appointment because of diarrhea that has lasted for 2 weeks. The nurse answering the phone tells Mrs. M to "stop taking all of her medications" until she is seen in the clinic.

1. Do you agree or disagree with the nurse's advice to Mrs. M? Why?

You have been working in the clinical agency for nearly 6 months. Recently you noticed a colleague having difficulty completing his assignments on time. He also has been late for work on at least three occasions. Today you see him move from one patient to the next without washing his hands.

1. What are your options in this situation?

2. Discuss the possible consequences of each option.

3. What would you do? Why is this the best approach?

(continued)

Table 11.2 *(continued)*

Your patient has had diarrhea and abdominal pain for 8 days. She is scheduled for a number of diagnostic tests. As you complete her health history, she asks to see her chart.

1. What would you say to this patient?
2. What principles guide your decision? Provide a rationale for your response.

Mrs. J brings her 8-year-old daughter, Laura, into the office for her annual visit. In reviewing the immunization record, the nurse notices that Laura never received the second dose of MMR (measles, mumps, rubella). The nurse tells the mother not to worry. Laura can get the second dose when she is 11 or 12 years old.

1. Do you agree or disagree with the RN's advice to the mother? Provide a rationale for your decision.

Critical Thinking

Read the following statements: One in three adults and one in five adolescents are overweight. Being overweight is prevalent among certain racial and ethnic groups.

1. What additional information do you need before identifying the implications of this statement for your community?
2. Why is this information important?

Mr. J is developmentally delayed but has been able to live alone with the help of a neighbor. The neighbor, however, is moving. The neighbor calls your clinic and asks if someone can help Mr. J.

1. What are your options in this situation?
2. What critical information is needed before you decide what to do?

The owners of two home health care agencies in your community have complained that measures to decrease costs in the hospital have done nothing more than shift the costs to them.

1. What do you think about this statement?

(continued)

Table 11.2 *(continued)*

---

2. Examine this statement from the point of view of the hospital administrators and their attempt to control costs and the point of view of the home health administrators and their concerns about costs.

3. How would you revise this statement, if at all?

The Social Policy Statement says that "the presence of illness does not preclude health nor does optimal health preclude illness" (American Nurses Association, 1995, p. 4).

1. What is the reasoning behind this statement?

2. Describe another point of view and develop a rationale to support it.

CASE STUDY

A case study provides an actual patient situation or a hypothetical one for students to analyze and arrive at varied decisions. Case studies are typically longer and more comprehensive than in case method, providing background data about the patient, family history, and other information for a more complete picture. For this reason, students can analyze case studies in greater depth than with case method and present a more detailed rationale for their analysis. In their critique of the case study, students can describe the concepts and theories that guided their analysis, how they used them in understanding the case, and the literature they reviewed. Examples of case studies are presented in Table 11.3.

Fuszard (1995) suggested that after analyzing the case study, the teacher and students review the theoretical issues involved in the case to promote application to future clinical situations. Case studies may be integrated in clinical courses throughout the curriculum to assist students in applying concepts and theories from class to patient situations of increasing complexity.

Su, Masoodi, Kopp, and Klonowski (1998) described an infusion approach using case studies for teaching critical thinking. The basic premise of this strategy is to promote the development of thinking skills among students using case studies, progressing from a modeling of the thought process by the teacher to thinking by the students themselves. Using a case history and thinking map to guide the thought process, the

Table 11.3 Examples of Case Studies

Ms. Stone, a community health nurse, visits Carol, who was sent home from the hospital 1 day after the normal delivery of her first child. A 1-day postpartum stay was the policy of the hospital based on insurance reimbursement policies. Carol was given instructions for care of the newborn and herself by the hospital nurse, and it was agreed that her mother and her husband would help with the new infant.

Ms. Stone calls to make an appointment to visit Carol and her baby. She is told by Carol's mother that the infant, who was being breast-fed, was the "best baby on earth." The grandmother also says that the infant never cries and never wakes up for a feeding during the night. Ms. Stone asks her to elaborate on her description of the infant. The grandmother says the infant appears more olive-skinned than in the hospital. Ms. Stone asks if she can visit within the next hour. The nurse finds the infant extremely jaundiced and dehydrated.

1. What are the possible problems the infant might be experiencing? Provide a rationale.
2. What should Ms. Stone do first? Why is this important?
3. List information in the case about the infant that is significant. What is the relationship of this information to the problems you identified?
4. Select one family theory and analyze the case using this theory.

Note. From *Community Health Nursing: An Alliance for Health* (p. 9) by M. Klainberg, S. Holzemer, M. Leonard, and J. Arnold, 1998, New York: McGraw-Hill. Copyright 1998 by McGraw-Hill. Adapted with permission.

David, age 24 years, was driving home late at night when he lost control of his car and hit a tree. On impact his head hit the windshield. A witness to the accident stated that David was unconscious for at least 5 minutes but was awake when the paramedics arrived on the scene at 3:00 A.M. On arrival to the emergency department, David was awake and restless with little memory of the accident. He was slightly combative with the staff. A small laceration was observed on his left temple. Skull x-rays identified a left-sided temporal fracture. Vital signs were:

(continued)

Table 11.3 *(continued)*

BP   120/80
HR   88 bpm
Respirations   22/minute
Temperature   36.6°C (97.8°F)

David was admitted to the medical-surgical unit for observation. He remained alert and oriented throughout the night with no changes noted in his neurologic status. However, at 7:00 A.M., David was very irritable and did not know the date or time. By 8:00 A.M. he became drowsy and was mumbling incoherently. The physician on call was notified, and a computed tomography (CT) scan was ordered, which revealed a left-sided epidural hematoma.

1. Describe the pathophysiology of an epidural hematoma.

2. What is the classic clinical picture of epidural hematoma? How does this compare to David's condition?

3. In the event that the epidural hematoma progresses to uncal hernation, what clinical manifestations may be observed?

4. Discuss options for surgical intervention for David.

5. What nursing or patient actions can result in an increased intracranial pressure? Why?

6. What pharmacologic agents might be used to decrease intracranial pressure and cerebral edema for a patient with an epidural hematoma?

7. Describe nursing responsibilities for assessing and monitoring David's neurological status.

8. What nursing interventions would be important for David's care? Include a rationale for each intervention.

From "Epidural Hematoma" by L. S. P. Smith and C. Alexander in *Review of Critical Care Nursing: Case Studies and Applications* (pp. 216, 218), by S. D. Melander, 1996, Philadelphia: W. B. Saunders. Copyright (c) 1996 by W. B. Saunders. Adapted with permission.

---

teacher begins by modeling critical thinking step by step through a case. Students then practice their thinking following this demonstration (Su et al., 1998). For example, after reading a case study about a family with a chronically ill child, the teacher models how to find cues in the case situation, identify which cues from family members are significant, and draw inferences from them. Students then identify other cues and generate new inferences in small groups.

DEVELOPING CASES

Case method and study have two components: a case situation for review and analysis by the student and questions to answer about the case or from its analysis. In case method, the actual situations described are typically short and geared to specific objectives to be met.

Case studies include background information about the patient, family history, and complete assessment data to provide a comprehensive description of the patient or clinical situation. Goodman (1997) recommended that when used for orientation of new staff, the cases should be based on examples that orientees are likely to encounter in the clinical area. Goodman (1997) developed integrated cases for orientation. The case description includes psychosocial history, medical history, presenting condition, ethical issues, safety concerns, interpersonal situations, and age-specific implications if relevant. Related psychomotor skills also can be identified to highlight their use with the patient described in the case study. For example, a case study on the care of an elderly patient with a hip fracture might include a list of these skills: positioning, mobility exercises, use of splints, how to set up an overhead frame and trapeze, and planning for discharge, including equipment needed for home care (Goodman, 1997).

The case should provide enough information for analysis without directing the students' thinking in a particular direction. The case may be developed first, then the questions, or the teacher may draft the questions first, then develop the case to present the clinical situation.

The questions developed for the case are the key to its effective use. They should be geared to the outcomes to be met. For instance, if the intent of the case study is to analyze laboratory data, apply physiological principles, and use concepts of pathophysiology for the analysis, then the questions need to relate to each of these. Similarly, if the goal is to improve problem-solving skills, then the questions should ask about the problems described in the case, any possible alternate problems, the supporting data, the additional data needed, and the possible solutions. With most cases, questions should be included that focus on the underlying thought process used to arrive at an answer rather than the answer alone.

Case method and study assist students in relating course content to clinical practice and integrating different concepts and theories in a particular client situation. Neill, Lachat, and Taylor-Panek (1997) developed case studies for use throughout a clinical course. Each case consists of a description of a patient at different points in time, for instance, from admission through discharge. Questions developed for the case focus on critical thinking and use of knowledge in clinical practice. Cases are analyzed in small groups.

A variation of case study is unfolding cases in which the clinical situation is ever-changing, thereby creating a simulation for students to critique. In the model by Glendon and Ulrich (1997), three paragraphs are developed. The first paragraph sets the stage of the case, including background information about the patient and others, a description of the clinical situation, and questions for discussion by students. After the initial analysis of the case by the students, the next paragraph is revealed, changing the scenario in some way. Once again, students critique the new information and answer related questions. After reading the last paragraph, students complete a reflective writing exercise in which they project future learning needs and share individual feelings and reactions to the case.

In designing cases to promote problem solving, develop a case that asks students to

- identify patient and other problems apparent in the case
- suggest alternate problems that might be possible if more information was available and identify the information needed
- identify relevant and irrelevant information in the case
- propose different approaches that might be used
- identify advantages and disadvantages of each approach
- select the best approaches for solving problems in the case situation
- provide a theoretical rationale for these approaches
- identify gaps in the literature and research as related to the case
- evaluate the effectiveness of interventions
- plan alternate interventions based on analysis of the case

An example of a case for problem solving is the following:

Ms. G, a 56-year-old patient admitted for shortness of breath and chest pain, is scheduled for a cardiac catheterization. She has been crying on-and-off for the last hour. When the nurse attempts to talk to her, Ms. G says, "Don't worry about me. I'm just tired."

1. What is one problem in this situation that needs to be solved?
2. What assumptions about Ms. G did you make in identifying this problem?
3. What additional information would you collect from the patient and her medical records before intervening? Why is this information important?

Cases for decision making may be developed in two ways. The case may present a clinical situation up to the point of a decision, then ask students to critique the case and arrive at a decision. Or the case may describe a situation and decision, then ask whether students agree or disagree with it. For both of these types, the questions should lead the students through the decision-making process, and students should include a rationale for their responses.

For decision making, develop a case that asks students to

- identify the decisions needed in the case
- identify information in the case that is critical for arriving at a decision
- specify additional data needed for a decision
- examine alternative decisions possible and the consequences of each
- arrive at a decision and provide a rationale for it.

An example of a case intended for decision making is the following:

The nurse manager on the midnight shift in a large hospital assigns a nurse new to the unit to work with Ms. P, an experienced RN. Ms. P, however, is irate that she needs to orient a new nurse when she is "so busy" herself. Ms. P tells the new nurse that she is too busy to work with her tonight. When learning this, the manager reassigns the new nurse to another RN.

1. Do you agree or disagree with the nurse manager's decision? Why?
2. Describe at least two strategies you could use in this situation. What are advantages and disadvantages of each?
3. How would you handle this situation?

Case method and study also meet critical thinking outcomes. For critical thinking:

Develop cases that:

Present an issue for analysis, a question to be answered that has multiple possibilities, or a complex problem to be solved.

Ask students to:

Analyze the case and provide a rationale for the thinking process they used for the analysis.

Examine the assumptions underlying their thinking.

Describe the evidence on which their reasoning was based.

Describe the concepts and theories they used for their analysis and *how* they applied to the case.

Have different and conflicting points of view.	Analyze the case from their own point of view, then analyze the case from a different point of view.
Present complex data for analysis.	Analyze the data and draw possible inferences given the data. Specify additional information needed and why this is important.
Present clinical situations that are unique and offer different perspectives.	Analyze the situation, identify multiple perspectives possible, and examine assumptions made about the situation that influenced thinking.
Describe ethical issues and dilemmas.	Propose alternative solutions and consequences of different approaches. Weigh alternatives and arrive at a decision. Critique an issue from a different point of view.

An example of a case for critical thinking is:

You are a nurse practitioner working in a middle school. S, a 16-year-old, comes to your office for nausea and vomiting. She feels "bloated." She confides in you that she is pregnant and asks you not to tell her parents.

1. What are your options at this time?
2. What would you do next? Why?
3. Choose another option that you listed with question 1. What are the advantages and disadvantages of that approach over yours?

Whiteside (1997) developed a critical thinking model for nursing that provides a framework for designing case studies. The model begins by having students list and prioritize current and potential problems, then progresses to determining if additional data are needed, examining the assumptions made, providing a rationale for the problem, identifying goals and methods of achieving them, predicting the effects of the methods, choosing a course of action, and identifying possible unexpected consequences of the action (p. 155).

The model provides a schema for developing the case and related questions. A case may be geared to any number of steps in the model or to reflect the entire model, from listing the problems through identifying unexpected consequences of actions planned for them. For example, the teacher may design a case to promote skill in (1) listing and prioritizing current and potential problems and (2) determining if additional data are needed, the first two steps in the model. The next case provides an example:

Mrs. B, 29 years old, is seen for her prenatal checkup. She is in her 24th week of pregnancy. The nurse practitioner notes swelling of the ankles and around Mrs. B's eyes. Mrs. B has not been able to wear her rings for a week because of swelling. Her blood pressure is 144/96.

1. What are the possible problems Mrs. B might be facing? List all possible problems given the above information.
2. What additional data should be collected at this time? Why?

Alternately, the same case might be used, but questions might focus on assumptions made about Mrs. B's symptoms, goals the nurse should set for Mrs. B, measures for meeting these goals, and different approaches to care that might be taken. Using the same case, the questions might be:

1. Name one possible problem for Mrs. B.
2. What assumptions did you make about Mrs. B's condition that led you to this problem?
3. Develop a goal of care for this patient.
4. List three actions to be taken at this time. Why is each of these important in Mrs. B's care?
5. What would you do first? Why?

GRAND ROUNDS

Grand rounds involve the observation and often interview of a patient or several patients in the clinical setting, focusing on a particular condition or treatment. They may be conducted for nursing personnel only or as an interdisciplinary activity. Rounds provide an opportunity to observe a patient with a specific condition, review assessment data, discuss interventions and their effectiveness, and make changes in the plan of care. They are valuable for examining issues facing patients and discussing ways of resolving them. In a survey of general surgical residency programs, Downing, Way, and Caniano (1997) found that 50% of the programs provided their instruction in ethics through grand rounds.

Depending on the objectives, grand rounds might include the following areas for discussion: review of relevant pathophysiology; background information about the patient; the patient's history, including reason for admission, past medical history, relevant test results, and family history; nursing diagnoses and care; interdisciplinary referrals; related research; and patient outcomes (Kreichelt & Spann, 1991; McLean, Meyer, Schafer, & Schroeder, 1994). In some instances, procedures might be demonstrated with the patient's permission.

Anderson-Loftin (1995) described student-led nursing rounds as an interactive, patient-centered strategy in which students discuss a concept related to the care of an individual patient. Students present the topic at the patient's bedside for discussion with the patient and family and for later analysis by the clinical group (p. 242). The students who are not conducting the rounds observe the interaction, ask questions, and share their own observations and insights.

Grand rounds enable students to

- identify patient problems and issues in clinical practice
- evaluate the effectiveness of nursing and interdisciplinary interventions
- share clinical knowledge with peers and identify gaps in own understanding
- develop new perspectives to care
- gain insight into other ways of meeting patient needs
- think critically about the nursing care they provide and that given by their peers
- dialogue about patient care and changes in nursing practice with peers and experts participating in the rounds.

Sedlak and Doheny (1998) described a clinical teaching strategy that used peer review during student-led rounds to promote critical thinking. At the end of each clinical day, groups of three to four students each conducted walking rounds in place of a postconference. Students first described briefly important physical and psychosocial assessment data and identified nursing diagnoses, interventions, and outcomes. Then they presented their patients to the group while their peers observed and asked questions, noting positive aspects of care and areas needing further clarification.

To facilitate the presentation of the patient and discussion for the purpose of critical thinking, Schumacher and Severson (1996) developed a guide for presenters that includes these steps:

1. State the purpose of selecting the case for grand rounds, such as the complexity of nursing care, innovations being used in care, and interdisciplinary interventions.

2. Provide an overview of critical data.
3. Analyze possible diagnoses.
4. Formulate and critique nursing diagnostic statements including assumptions, misleading associations, and relationship to the data.
5. Identify variables that influence achieving patient outcomes.
6. Discuss nursing actions, related literature and research, and factors that might interfere with recommended nursing actions.
7. Explore insights gained, comparing the patient to other similar patients, identifying alternate approaches, and identifying system limitations that might interfere with implementation of the nursing actions (p. 32).

Grand rounds may be conducted by an advanced practice nurse, a staff nurse, the teacher, the student, or another health professional. For student-led rounds, the teacher is responsible for confirming the plan with the patient. Patients should be assured of their right to refuse participation and should be comfortable to tell the student or teacher when they no longer want to continue with it.

Activities at the patient's bedside should begin with an introduction of the patient to the students, emphasizing the patient's contribution to student learning. If possible, the person conducting the rounds should include the patient and family in the discussion, seeking their perspective of the health problem and input into care. The teacher's role is that of consultant, clarifying information and assisting the student in keeping the discussion on the goals set for the rounds. The teacher should ask questions and discuss sensitive issues after the rounds are completed and out of the patient's presence.

SUMMARY

Case method and case study describe a clinical situation, developed around an actual or hypothetical patient, for student review and critique. In case method the case provided for analysis is generally shorter and more specific than in case study. Case studies are more comprehensive in nature, thereby presenting a complete picture of the patient and clinical situation.

With these clinical teaching methods, students apply concepts and theories to practice situations, identify actual and potential problems, propose varied approaches for solving them, weigh different decisions possible, and arrive at judgments as to the effectiveness of interventions. As such, case method and study provide experience for students in thinking through different client situations. They are valuable for promoting development of problem-solving, decision-making, and critical thinking skills.

Grand rounds involve the observation and often interview of a patient or several patients in the clinical setting, focusing on a particular condition or treatment. They may be conducted for nursing personnel only or as an interdisciplinary activity. Rounds provide an opportunity to observe a patient with a specific condition, review assessment data, discuss interventions and their effectiveness, and make changes in the plan of care. They also are valuable for examining issues facing patients and discussing ways of resolving them. Grand rounds, similar to case method and study, provide an opportunity for exploring patient problems and varied solutions, analyzing care and proposing new interventions, and gaining insight into different patient situations.

REFERENCES

American Nurses Association. (1995). *Nursing's social policy statement*. Washington, DC: Author.

Anderson-Loftin, W. (1995). Nursing rounds. In B. Fuszard, *Innovative teaching strategies in nursing* (2nd ed., pp. 242–253). Gaithersburg, MD: Aspen.

Downing, M. T., Way, D. P., & Caniano, D. A. (1997). Results of a national survey on ethics education in general surgery residency programs. *American Journal of Surgery, 174*(3), 364–368.

Facione, N. C., & Facione, P. (1996). Externalizing the critical thinking in knowledge development and clinical judgment. *Nursing Outlook, 44*, 129–136.

Fuszard, B. (1995). Case method. In B. Fuszard, *Innovative teaching strategies in nursing* (2nd ed., pp. 81–92). Gaithersburg, MD: Aspen.

Glendon, K., & Ulrich, D. L. (1997). Unfolding cases: An experiential learning model. *Nurse Educator, 22*(4), 15–18.

Goodman, D. (1997). Application of the critical pathway and integrated case teaching method to nursing orientation. *Journal of Continuing Education in Nursing, 28*, 205–210.

Kataoka-Yahiro, M., & Saylor, C. (1994). A critical thinking model for nursing judgment. *Journal of Nursing Education, 33*, 351–356.

Kreichelt, G., & Spann, K. (1991). Brief: Medical nursing grand rounds: Learning, sharing, caring. *Journal of Continuing Education in Nursing, 22*, 35.

McLean, P., Meyer, K., Schafer, B., & Schroeder, B. (1994). Nursing grand rounds facilitate staff development. *Oncology Nursing Forum, 21*, 600.

Neill, K. M., Lachat, M. F., & Taylor-Panek, S. (1997). Enhancing critical thinking with case studies and nursing process. *Nurse Educator, 22*(2), 30–32.

Nitko, A. J. (1996). *Educational assessment of students* (2nd ed.). Englewood Cliffs, NJ: Prentice-Hall.

Oermann, M. H. (1997). Evaluating critical thinking in clinical practice. *Nurse Educator, 22*(5), 25–28.

———. (1998). How to assess critical thinking in clinical practice. *Dimensions of Critical Care Nursing, 17*, 322–327.

Oermann, M. H., & Gaberson, K. (1998). *Evaluation and testing in nursing education.* New York: Springer.

Schön, D. A. (1990). *Educating the reflective practitioner.* San Francisco: Jossey-Bass.

Schumacher, J., & Severson, A. (1996). Building bridges for future practice: An innovative approach to foster critical thinking. *Journal of Nursing Education, 35,* 31–33.

Sedlak, C. A. (1997). Critical thinking of beginning baccalaureate nursing students during their first clinical course. *Journal of Nursing Education, 36,* 11–18.

Sedlak, C. A., & Doheny, M. O. (1998). Peer review through clinical rounds. *Nurse Educator, 23*(5), 42–45.

Su, W. M., Masoodi, J., Kopp, M., & Klonowski, E. (1998). Infusing teaching thinking skills into subject-area instruction. *Nurse Educator, 23*(4), 27–30.

Whiteside, C. (1997). A model for teaching critical thinking in the clinical setting. *Dimensions of Critical Care Nursing, 16,* 152–162.

12

Clinical Conference and Discussion

Clinical conferences and discussions with learners provide a means of sharing information, developing problem-solving and critical thinking skills, and learning how to collaborate with others in a group. Discussion is an exchange of ideas for a specific purpose; clinical conferences are a form of group discussion that focus on some aspect of clinical practice. Teachers and students engage in many discussions in planning, carrying out, and evaluating the clinical learning activities. Similarly, there are varied types of clinical conferences for use in teaching. Effective conferences and discussions require an understanding of their goals, the types of questions for encouraging the exchange of ideas and higher level thinking, and the roles of the teacher and students.

DISCUSSION

Discussions between teacher and student, preceptor and orientee, and nurse manager and staff occur frequently but do not always promote learning. Often these discussions involve the teacher "telling" the learner what to do or not to do in regard to patient care. Discussions, though, should be an exchange of ideas through which the teacher, by asking open-ended questions and supporting learner responses, encourages students to arrive at their own decisions or to engage in self-assessment about clinical practice. Discussions are not intended to be an "exchange" of the teacher's ideas *to* the students. In a discussion both teacher and student actively participate in sharing ideas and considering alternate perspectives.

Discussions give learners an opportunity to interact with one another, critique each other's ideas, and learn from others. The teacher is a resource for students, giving immediate feedback and further instruction as needed. Discussions provide a forum for students to express ideas, explore feelings associated with their clinical practice, clarify values and ethical dilemmas, and learn to interact in a group format. These outcomes are not as easily met in a large group setting. Over a period of time, students learn to collaborate with peers in working toward solving clinical problems.

Creating a Climate for Discussion

An important role of the teacher is to develop a climate in which students are comfortable discussing concepts and issues without fear that the ideas expressed will affect the teacher's evaluation of their performance and subsequent clinical grade. Along the same line, discussions between preceptor and orientee and between manager and staff should be carried out in an atmosphere in which nurses feel comfortable to express their own opinions and ideas and to question others' assumptions (Oermann, 1998). Discussions are not intended for summative evaluation; they serve only a formative purpose, providing feedback to learners individually or in a small group. Without this climate for exchanging ideas, though, discussions cannot be carried out effectively because students fear that their comments may influence their clinical evaluation and grade, or for nurses, their performance ratings.

The teacher sets an atmosphere in which listening, respect for others' comments and ideas, and openness to new perspectives are valued (Schell, 1998). Learners need to be free to discuss their ideas and uncertainties, offer their opinions, and express alternate views. Without support from the teacher, students will not participate freely in the discussion, nor will they be willing to examine controversial points of view, critique different perspectives to care and decisions, or share misunderstandings with the teacher and peers.

Students who perceive their teachers as being supportive are more likely to ask questions (Karabenick & Sharma, 1994). Studies on teacher effectiveness highlight the importance of this interpersonal relationship between teacher and students. Important characteristics of effective teaching, among others, are conveying confidence in and respect for students, being honest and direct, and encouraging students to ask questions and participate freely in discussions (Bergman & Gaitskill, 1990; Oermann, 1996).

Guidelines for Discussion

Discussions may be carried out individually with learners or in a small group. The size of the group for a discussion may range from 2 to 10 people. Any larger group makes it difficult for each person to participate.

The teacher is responsible for planning the discussion to meet the clinical objectives and keeping the interactions focused on these outcomes. An effective teacher keeps the discussion focused; avoids talking too much, with students in a passive role; and avoids side-tracking. While the teacher may initiate the discussion, the interaction needs to revolve around the students, not the teacher. Students may be prompted, but the teacher should avoid thinking for the students and asking questions with specific answers in mind (Meyers, 1986). Rephrasing students' questions for them to answer suggests that the teacher has confidence in the students' ability to arrive at answers and provides opportunities to develop critical thinking skills.

The teacher also should be aware of the environment in which the discussion takes place. Chairs should be arranged in a configuration, such as a circle, semi-circle, or U-shape, that encourages interaction. For some discussions, students may be divided into pairs or other smaller groups. Table 12.1 summarizes the roles of the teacher and students in clinical discussions.

Guidelines for planning a discussion and effectively using it in the practice setting follow:

- Identify the outcomes and goals to be achieved in the discussion considering the time frame.
- Plan questions for structured discussions ahead of time. They may be written for the teacher only or also for students. If not written, plan for the direction of the discussion and important content to be included prior to beginning it.
- Plan *how* the discussion will be carried out. Will all students in the clinical group participate, or will they be divided into smaller groups or pairs, then share the results of their individual discussions with the clinical group?
- Sequence questions depending on the desired outcomes of the discussion.
- Ask open-ended questions that encourage multiple perspectives and different lines of thinking.
- Think about how the questions are phrased before asking them.
- Ask questions to the group as a whole or ask for volunteers to respond. If questions are directed to a specific learner, be sensitive to his or her comfort in responding and do not create undue stress for the student. If this occurs, the teacher should provide prompts or cues for responding.

Table 12.1 Roles of Teacher and Student in Discussion

Teacher

Plans discussion

Presents problem, issue, case for analysis

Develops questions for discussion

Facilitates discussion and encourages students to participate

Develops and maintains atmosphere for open discussion of ideas and
issues

Keeps time

Avoids side-tracking

Provides feedback

Student

Prepares for discussion

Participates actively in discussion

Works collaboratively with group members to arrive at solutions and
decisions

Examines different points of view

Is willing to modify own view and perspective to reach group consensus

Teacher and Student

Summarize outcomes of discussion

Relate discussion to theory and research

Identify implications of discussion for other clinical situations

- Wait 3 to 5 seconds between the question and request for a response
  (Schell, 1998).
- Give students time to answer the questions. If no one responds, try
  rephrasing the question.
- Reinforce students' answers indicating why they were appropriate
  or not for the question.
- Give nonverbal and verbal feedback to encourage student participation without overusing it.
- Avoid interrupting the learner even if errors are noted in the line
  of thinking or information. Correct these errors when the learner
  is finished.

- Correct students' errors in thinking and responding without belittling them. Focus on the answer and errors in reasoning, not on the student.
- Listen carefully to students' responses and make notes to remember points made in the discussion. Tell students ahead of time that any notes are for use only during the discussion, not for student evaluation or other purposes. Destroy the notes so students are assured of their freedom to respond in discussions.
- If further discussion is needed, ask follow-up questions.
- Assess your own skill in directing discussions and identify areas for improvement.

Discussions may begin with questions raised by the teacher or by students directed toward the learning outcomes or may be integrated with other instructional methods, such as case scenarios, simulations, games, role play, and media clips. Case scenarios, for instance, may be critiqued and then discussed by students in a clinical conference. Fuszard (1995) described a method in which cases are distributed to students prior to clinical practice; students then review related literature and identify issues in the case. The clinical group discusses the case, identifies problems and solutions, and makes decisions, integrating the literature in the discussion. Or students may play a game and complete a role play exercise, followed by discussion. Media clips provide an effective format for presenting a clinical situation for analysis and discussion.

Purposes of Discussion

In a discussion the teacher has an opportunity to ask carefully selected questions about students' thinking and the rationale used for arriving at decisions and positions about issues. Discussions may be impromptu or planned by the teacher.

Discussions promote several types of learning, depending on the goals and structure: developing problem-solving, decision-making, and critical thinking skills; debriefing clinical experiences; developing cooperative learning and group process skills; assessing own learning; and developing oral communication skills. Every discussion will not necessarily promote each of these learning outcomes; the teacher should be clear as to the intent of the discussion so it may be geared to the particular outcomes to be achieved. For instance, discussions for critical thinking require carefully selected questions that examine alternate possibilities and "what if" types of questions. This same questioning, however, may not be necessary if the goal is to develop cooperative learning or group process skills.

DEVELOPING COGNITIVE SKILLS

An important purpose of discussion is to promote development of prob-lem-solving, decision-making, and critical thinking skills. Discussions are effective because they provide an opportunity for the teacher to gear the questioning toward each of these skills, either by asking questions during or planning them prior to the discussion.

There are many ways for discussions to be directed toward develop-ment of problem-solving, decision-making, and critical thinking skills. Not all discussions, though, lead to these higher levels of thinking. The key to these discussions are the questions asked by the teacher or discussed among students that encourage them to examine alternate perspectives and points of view in a given situation and to provide a rationale for their decisions and positions about issues.

In these discussions, students may be given a hypothetical or real clin-ical situation involving a patient, family, or community to critique and identify potential problems. Students may discuss possible decisions, rea-sons underlying each decision, consequences and implications of options they considered as part of their decision making, and different points of view in the situation. Alternately, a situation may be presented for students to identify issues to be solved, assumptions underlying their thinking, mul-tiple perspectives possible in the situation, and different approaches for resolving the issue. Table 12.2 presents strategies for directing discussions toward development of problem-solving, decision-making, and critical thinking skills.

DEBRIEFING CLINICAL EXPERIENCES

Discussions provide an opportunity for students to report on their clinical learning activities; describe and analyze the care they provided to patients, families, and communities; and share their feelings and perceptions about their clinical experiences. In these discussions students receive feedback from peers and the teacher about alternate decisions and approaches pos-sible. Debriefing clinical experiences allows students to share feelings and perceptions about their patients and clinical situations in a comfortable environment. Stokes (1998) viewed this type of clinical discussion as essen-tial for developing support systems for students. Issues with patients, staff, and others may be examined and critiqued by the group. Discussions of this nature provide a an opportunity for the teacher to help students exam-ine their decisions and learn from others. Typically, this debriefing is held as a postclinical conference, at the end of a clinical day or following com-pletion of specific clinical activities.

Table 12.2 Discussions for Cognitive Skill Development

Ask students to:

  Identify problems and issues in a real or hypothetical clinical situation

  Identify alternate problems possible

  Assess the problem further

  Differentiate relevant and irrelevant information for problem or issue
    being discussed

  Discuss own point of view and those of others

  Examine assumptions they made and those of other students

  Identify different solutions, courses of action, and consequences of each

  Consider both positive and negative consequences

  Compare possible alternatives and defend why they would choose one
    particular solution or action over another

  Take a position about an issue and provide a rationale both for and
    against that position

  Identify their own biases, values, and beliefs that influence their thinking

  Identify obstacles to solving a problem

  Evaluate the effectiveness of interventions and approaches to solving
    problems

DEVELOPING COOPERATIVE LEARNING SKILLS

Group discussions are effective for promoting cooperative learning skills. Cooperative learning is an interactive teaching strategy that fosters critical thinking and promotes individual accountability for learning in a group format (Glendon & Ulrich, 1992). Students work cooperatively in groups to meet predetermined goals. The outcomes of their discussions are solutions to problems and completion of the tasks assigned by the teacher. Cooperative learning strategies differ from traditional group work in that group rewards and incentives may be offered to increase cooperation in the group, and students are held individually accountable for the quality of their participation (Glendon & Ulrich, 1992).

Discussions using cooperative learning strategies begin with the teacher planning the discussion, presenting a task to be completed by the group or a problem to be solved, developing an environment for open discussion, and facilitating the discussion. In this type of discussion, the teacher identifies a clinical problem to be solved and plans the activities of the group. Students work cooperatively in groups to propose solutions, complete the tasks, and present the results of their discussions to the rest of the students.

There are different techniques for promoting cooperative learning as an outcome of discussions. Each student may complete the task individually, then report his or her findings to the clinical group; students may work in pairs, then share the results of their thinking to the group; or the teacher may divide the students into smaller groups of about four to six students each to facilitate discussion and problem solving. With each of these strategies, though, the teacher monitors the discussion and after students report to the group, clarifies the information presented, reemphasizes the important content to be learned, and assists students in evaluating their group process skills.

ASSESSING OWN LEARNING

Discussions provide a means for students to assess their own learning, identify gaps in their understanding, and learn from others in a non-threatening environment. Students can ask questions of the group and use the teacher and peers as resources for their learning. If the teacher is effective in developing an atmosphere for open discussion, students, in turn, will share their feelings, concerns, and questions as a beginning to their continued development.

DEVELOPING ORAL COMMUNICATION SKILLS

The ability to present ideas orally, as well as in written form, is an important outcome to be achieved by students in clinical courses (Applegate, 1998; Oermann, 1994). Discussions provide experience for students in presenting ideas to a group, explaining concepts clearly, handling questions raised by others, and refining presentation style. Participation in a discussion requires formulating ideas and presenting them logically to the group. Students also may make formal presentations to the clinical group as a way of developing their oral communication skills. They may lead a discussion and present on a specific topic related to the clinical objectives. Discussion provides an opportunity for peers and the teacher to give feedback to students on how well students communicated their ideas to others.

Table 12.3 presents an evaluation form that students may use to rate the quality of presentations and provide feedback on ability to lead a group discussion. This form is not intended for summative, or grading, purposes, but instead is designed for giving feedback to students following a presentation to the clinical group.

Table 12.3 Evaluation Form for Rating Presentations in Conferences

Name _____

Title of Presentation _____

Rate each of the behaviors listed below. Circle the appropriate number and give feedback to the presenter in the space provided.

Behavior	Rating				
	1 Little	2	3	4	5 Much
Leadership Role in Conference					
1. Leads the group in discussion of ideas	1	2	3	4	5
2. Encourages active participation of peers in conference	1	2	3	4	5
3. Encourages open discussion of ideas	1	2	3	4	5
4. Helps group synthesize ideas presented	1	2	3	4	5

Comments:

Quality of Content Presented					
5. Prepares objectives for presentation that reflect clinical goals	1	2	3	4	5
6. Presents content that relates to objectives and is relevant for students' clinical practice	1	2	3	4	5
7. Presents content that is accurate and up-to-date	1	2	3	4	5
8. Presents content that reflects theory and research	1	2	3	4	5

Comments:

(continued)

Table 12.3 *(continued)*

Quality of Presentation

9. Organizes and presents material logically	1	2	3	4	5
10. Explains ideas clearly	1	2	3	4	5
11. Plans presentation considering time demands and needs of clinical group	1	2	3	4	5
12. Emphasizes key points	1	2	3	4	5
13. Encourages students to ask questions	1	2	3	4	5
14. Answers students' questions accurately	1	2	3	4	5
15. Supports alternate viewpoints and encourages their discussion	1	2	3	4	5
16. Is enthusiastic	1	2	3	4	5

Comments:

LEVEL OF QUESTIONS

The level of questions asked in any discussion is the key to directing it toward the intended learning outcomes. In most clinical discussions the goal is to avoid a predominance of factual questions and focus instead on clarifying and higher level questions. There are different frameworks, such as Bloom's and Ebel's taxonomies, that may be used to sequence questions in a discussion with an individual student or clinical group.

The taxonomy of the cognitive domain, related to knowledge and intellectual skills, was developed by Bloom (Bloom, Englehart, Furst, Hill, & Krathwohl, 1956) many years ago but is still of value today for developing objectives and test items and for leveling questions. Learning in the cognitive domain includes the acquisition of facts and specific information; concepts, theories, and principles underlying nursing practice; and cognitive skills of problem solving, decision making, clinical judgment, and critical thinking (Oermann & Gaberson, 1998). The cognitive taxonomy includes six levels that increase in complexity: knowledge, comprehension, application, analysis, synthesis, and evaluation. These levels are arranged in a hierarchy, with recall of specific facts and information being the least complex level of learning and evaluating clinical situations and making judgments, the most complex.

The cognitive taxonomy is useful in asking questions in a discussion or planning questions for student response, because it levels them along a continuum from ones requiring only recall of facts to higher level questions requiring synthesis of knowledge and evaluation. The teacher may begin by asking students factual questions, then progress to questions that are answered based on a comprehension and understanding of the facts, the use of concepts and theories, analysis, synthesis of material from different sources, and evaluation.

A description and sample questions for each of the six levels of the cognitive taxonomy follow. Sample words for use in developing questions at each level are presented in Table 12.4.

1. Knowledge: Recall of facts and specific information; memorization of facts.
   "Define the term percussion."
   "What is this type of arrhythmia called?"

2. Comprehension: Understanding; ability to describe and explain.
   "Tell me about your patient's shortness of breath."
   "What does this potassium level indicate?"

3. Application: Use of information in a *new or novel* situation; ability to use knowledge in a new situation.
   "Why are these interventions appropriate from a family stress perspective?"
   "Tell me about Mr. S's problems and related pathophysiological changes. Why are each of these changes important for you to monitor?"

4. Analysis: Ability to break down material into component parts and identify the relationships among them.
   "What effects does the organizational structure of the hospital and its home care agency have on services for patients and the nurse's role?"
   "What assumptions did you make about this family that influenced your decisions? What are alternate approaches to consider?"

5. Synthesis: Ability to develop new ideas and materials; combining elements to form a new product.
   "Tell me about your plan to improve prenatal care for the women

Table 12.4 Question Classification

Level	Types of question	Sample words for questions
1. Knowledge	*Recall* Questions that can be answered by recall of facts and previously learned information	Define, identify, list, name, recall
2. Comprehension	*Understand* Questions that can be answered by explaining and describing	Describe, differentiate, draw conclusions, explain, give examples of, interpret, tell me in your own words
3. Application	*Use* Questions that require use of information in *new* situations	Apply, relate, use
4. Analysis	*Divide into component parts* Questions that ask students to break down material into its component parts, to analyze data and clinical situations	Analyze, compare, contrast, detect, identify reasons and assumptions, provide evidence to support conclusions, relate
5. Synthesis	*Develop new ideas and products* Questions or directives that ask students to develop new ideas, plans, products	Construct, create, design, develop, propose a plan, suggest a new approach
6. Evaluation	*Evaluate* Questions that require students to make a judgment based on criteria	Appraise, assess, critique, evaluate, judge, select

who come to your clinic. Why is your plan better than the existing services?"
"Develop a care plan for patients receiving home care after hip replacement."

6. Evaluation: Judgments about value based on internal and external criteria; evaluating extent to which materials meet predetermined criteria.
"Take a position for or against closing the clinic and shifting patients to the other center. Provide a rationale for your position."
"What is the impact on patients and families of providing one fewer home care visit?"

Questions for discussions should be sequenced from low-level to high-level, beginning with recall questions to assess learners' knowledge of relevant facts, concepts, and theories, then asking them to explain their answers further. The taxonomy provides a schema for progressing to questions at higher levels of learning (Wink, 1993). These higher level questions cannot be answered by memory alone. An example of a progression of questions using the taxonomy follows:

Knowledge:	"Define the gate control theory of pain."
Comprehension:	"Explain the physiological mechanisms underlying the gate control theory of pain."
Application:	"Tell me about an intervention you are using for your patient and how its use and effectiveness may be explained by the gate control theory."
Analysis:	"Your patient seems more agitated near the end of the shift. What additional data have you collected? What are possible reasons for this response?"
Synthesis:	"Develop a pain management plan for your patient now and for his discharge home."
Evaluation:	"You indicated that your patient's pain continues to increase. What alternate pain interventions do you propose? Why would these interventions be more effective?"

Another taxonomy that might also be used to level questions in a discussion is one by Ebel (1965). Ebel's taxonomy has seven categories for developing questions:

1. Terminology
2. Factual information
3. Explanation

4. Calculation
5. Prediction
6. Recommended action
7. Evaluation.

These levels are hierarchical, similar to Bloom's taxonomy, and provide a guide for asking questions at different levels of complexity. Lower level questions deal with definitions and recalling facts, leading to more complex questions on recommending actions to take and evaluating clinical situations.

Research suggests that teachers by nature do not ask higher level questions of students. Typically, the questions asked in a discussion tend to focus on recall and comprehension rather than higher levels of thinking (Craig & Page, 1981; Oermann, 1996; Wang & Blumberg, 1983; Wink, 1995). While the intent of clinical discussions may be to improve analytical thinking, this goal will not be met with questions that are answered by memorization of facts and specific information. Careful questioning with attention to the level of questions asked enables students to apply previously acquired knowledge to a situation, analyze problems and solutions, and develop critical thinking and problem-solving skills, among other benefits (Wink, 1995).

Socratic Method

The Socratic method also may be used as a basis for discussion. Socratic questions raise issues for students to consider, require analytical thinking to respond, and promote critical thinking. Socratic questions are an effective strategy when students are puzzled about a patient's problem and approaches to use or are faced with a problematic area of thinking. Paul (1993) identified seven aims of Socratic questioning:

1. Raise basic issues
2. Probe beneath the surface
3. Pursue problematic areas of thought
4. Discover structure of own thinking
5. Develop sensitivity to clarity, accuracy, and relevance
6. Arrive at judgments through own reasoning
7. Identify claims, evidence, conclusions, questions-at-issue, assumptions, implications, and different points of view (Paul, 1993, p. 336).

Socratic questioning involves two phases: (1) systematic questioning and (2) drawing comparisons. In the first phase, systematic questioning, the teacher plans a series of questions that lead students along predetermined paths to rational thinking (Overholser, 1992). Socratic questions are open-ended, with multiple responses possible. Usually, no one answer is correct. Questions ask students to consider different alternatives and varied points of view and to defend their choices.

In the second phase, questions focus on making comparisons across patients and to generalize learning from one patient and clinical situation to others. Examples of questions in this phase are "How are these assessments similar? Different?" "What patterns do you find in the data?" "What are similarities in nursing interventions for Mrs. S and your patient last week? In what ways does your nursing care differ and why?" One outcome of this line of questioning is to increase students' understanding of difficult concepts by having them arrive at a general understanding of a problem and solution that is applicable to other possible clinical scenarios (Oermann, 1997; Overholser, 1992).

Another model for carrying out Socratic questions in a discussion was developed by Paul (1993). This model provides a taxonomy of questions for the teacher to use for Socratic discussions:

- Questions of clarification
- Questions that probe assumptions
- Questions that probe reasons and evidence
- Questions about differing viewpoints or perspectives
- Questions that probe implications and consequences.

Table 12.5 gives sample questions in each category, based on Paul's (1993) taxonomy, that the teacher might use in clinical discussions.

CLINICAL CONFERENCES

Clinical conferences are discussions held in the clinical setting in which students share information about a client, lead others in discussions about clinical practice, present ideas in a group format, and give formal presentations to the group. Some clinical conferences involve other disciplines and provide necessary experience in working with other health professionals in planning and evaluating patient care. Conferences serve the same goals as any discussion: developing problem-solving, decision-making, and critical thinking skills; debriefing clinical experiences; developing cooperative learning and group process skills; assessing own learning; and developing oral communication skills. Guidelines for conducting clinical conferences are the same as for discussion and therefore are not repeated here.

There are many types of clinical conferences. *Preclinical conferences* are small group discussions that precede clinical learning activities. In pre-

Table 12.5 Socratic Questions

Clarification Questions

- Tell me about your client's condition/problems/needs.
- What is the most important client/family/community problem? Why?
- What do you mean when you say _____?
- Give me an example of _____.
- How does this new information relate to our earlier discussion of the family's care?

Questions to Probe Assumptions

- You seem to be assuming that your client's responses are due to _____. Tell me more about your thinking here.
- What assumptions have you made about _____?
- On what data have you based your decisions? Why?
- Your decisions about this client/family/community are based on your assumptions that _____. Is this always the case? Why or why not?

Questions to Probe Reasons

- How do you know that _____? What are other possible reasons for _____?
- Tell me why _____.
- What would you do if _____? Why?
- Is there a reason to question this information? decision? approach? Why?

Questions on Differing Perspectives

- What are other possibilities? alternatives?
- How might the client/family view this situation? Does anyone (in the clinical group) view this differently? Why?
- Tell me about different interventions that might be possible and why each one would be appropriate.
- What are other ways of approaching the staff?

Questions on Consequences

- If this occurs, then what would you expect to happen next? Why?
- What are the consequences of each of these possible approaches? What would you do in this situation and why?
- What would be the effect of ———— on the community?
- If this is true, then what?

Note. From Oermann, M. H. (1997). Evaluating critical thinking in clinical practice. *Nurse Educator, 22*(5), 25–28. Copyright 1997 by Lippincott, Williams, & Wilkins. Reprinted with permission.

clinical conferences students ask questions about their clinical learning activities, seek clarification about their clients' care and other aspects of clinical practice, and share concerns with the teacher and with peers. Preclinical conferences assist students in identifying patient problems, planning care, and evaluating its effectiveness; they prepare students for their clinical activities. An important role of the teacher in preclinical conferences is to assure that students have the essential knowledge and competencies to complete their clinical activities. In many instances the teacher needs to instruct students further and fill in the gaps in students' learning. Preclinical conferences may be conducted on a one-to-one basis with students or as a clinical group.

Postclinical conferences are held at the conclusion of clinical learning activities. Postclinical conferences provide a forum for discussing the clinical activities, analyzing clinical situations, expressing feelings, developing support systems among the students (Stokes, 1998), and achieving the other goals of discussion presented earlier. Postclinical conferences also may be used for peer review and critiquing each other's work. They are not intended, however, as substitutes for classroom instruction, with the teacher lecturing and presenting new content to students. A similar problem often occurs with guest speakers who treat the conference as a class, lecturing to students about their area of expertise rather than encouraging group discussion.

Issue conferences involve group discussion of issues associated with clinical practice, professional issues, and cultural, social, economic, and political issues (Reilly & Oermann, 1992). These conferences may focus on nursing practice only or involve other disciplines.

Interdisciplinary conferences provide an opportunity for collaborative planning and decision making about a patient's care, examining issues in the clinical setting that cross disciplines, and jointly planning approaches to solve client and other problems.

Critical incident conferences are discussions in which details of significant incidents in practice are explored by the group (Brookfield, 1995). In a critical incident conference, a single incident or event is presented to the clinical group for problem solving. The teacher or a student describes briefly an event that occurred in clinical practice that requires further analysis. The incident may be presented in written form or described orally for the group.

Through group discussion, students ask questions about the incident to gather sufficient information to identify the problem. Discussion then focuses on alternate approaches that might be used, varied decisions possible, and consequences of them. In this phase of the conference, students may identify individually the approaches they would take, then defend their choices to the group. Or students may work in groups to decide collaboratively on actions to take. At the end of the conference, the teacher, or student who presented the incident, reports what actually occurred and clarifies any misunderstandings among the students.

Debates provide a forum for analyzing problems and issues in depth, analyzing opposing viewpoints, and developing and defending a position to be taken. In a debate students should provide a rationale for their decisions. Debates developed around clinical issues give students an opportunity to prepare an argument for or against a particular position and to take a stand on an issue.

SUMMARY

Discussions are an exchange of ideas in a small group format. Discussions provide a forum for students to express ideas, explore feelings associated with their clinical practice, clarify values and ethical dilemmas, and learn to interact in a group format. Over a period of time, students learn to collaborate with peers in working toward solving clinical problems.

The teacher is a resource for students. By asking open-ended questions and supporting learner responses, the teacher encourages students to arrive at their own decisions and to engage in self-assessment about clinical practice. The teacher develops a climate in which students are comfortable discussing concepts and issues without fear that the ideas expressed will affect the teacher's evaluation of their performance and subsequent clinical grade.

Discussions promote several types of learning: developing problem-solving, decision-making, and critical thinking skills; debriefing clinical experiences; developing cooperative learning and group process skills; assessing own learning; and developing oral communication skills. The level of questions asked in any discussion is the key to directing it toward the intended learning outcomes. In most clinical discussions the goal is to avoid a predominance of factual questions and focus instead on clarifying and higher level questions. Questions for student response may be leveled along a continuum from ones requiring only recall of facts to higher level questions requiring synthesis of knowledge and evaluation. There are different frameworks, such as Bloom's and Ebel's taxonomies, that may be used to sequence questions in a discussion with an individual student or clinical group.

The Socratic method also may be used as a basis for discussion. Socratic questions raise issues for students to consider, require analytical thinking to respond, and promote critical thinking. Socratic questioning involves two phases: (1) systematic questioning and (2) drawing comparisons. In the first phase, systematic questioning, the teacher plans a series of questions that lead students along predetermined paths to rational thinking. Questions ask students to consider different alternatives and varied points of view and to defend their choices. In the second phase, questions focus on making comparisons across patients and generalizing learning from one patient and clinical situation to others.

Clinical conferences are discussions held in the clinical setting in which students share information about a client, lead others in discussions about clinical practice, present ideas in a group format, and give presentations to the group. Some clinical conferences involve other disciplines and provide necessary experience in working with other health professionals in planning and evaluating patient care. Conferences serve the same goals as any discussion. There are many types of clinical conferences: preclinical conference, postclinical conference, issue conference, interdisciplinary conference, and debates.

REFERENCES

Applegate, M. H. (1998). Curriculum evaluation. In D. M. Billings & J. A. Halstead, *Teaching in nursing* (pp. 179–208). Philadelphia: Saunders.

Bergman, K., & Gaitskill, T. (1990). Faculty and student perceptions of effective clinical teachers: An extension study. *Journal of Professional Nursing, 6*(1), 33–44.

Bloom, B. S., Englehart, M. D., Furst, E. J., Hill, W. H., & Krathwohl, D. R. (1956). *Taxonomy of educational objectives. The classification of educational goals. Handbook I: Cognitive domain*. White Plains, NY: Longman.

Brookfield, S. D. (1995). *Becoming a critically reflective teacher*. San Francisco: Jossey–Bass.

Craig, J. L., & Page, G. (1981). The questioning skills of nursing instructors. *Journal of Nursing Education, 20*, 18–23.

Ebel, R. L. (1965). *Measuring educational achievement*. Englewood Cliffs, NJ: Prentice-Hall.

Fuszard, B. (1995). Case method. In B. Fuszard, *Innovative teaching strategies in nursing* (2nd ed., pp. 81–92). Gaithersburg, MD: Aspen.

Glendon, K., & Ulrich, D. (1992). Using cooperative learning strategies. *Nurse Educator, 17*(4), 37–40.

Karabenick, S. A., & Sharma, R. (1994). Perceived teacher support of student questioning in the college classroom: Its relation to student characteristics and role in the classroom questioning process. *Journal of Educational Psychology, 86*(1), 90–103.

Meyers, C. (1986). *Teaching students to think critically*. San Francisco: Jossey-Bass.

Oermann, M. H. (1994). Reforming nursing education for future practice. *Journal of Nursing Education, 33*, 215–219.

———. (1996). Research on teaching in the clinical setting. In K. Stevens (Ed.), *Review of research in nursing education* (Vol. 7, pp. 91–126). New York: National League for Nursing.

————. (1997). Evaluating critical thinking in clinical practice. *Nurse Educator, 22*(5), 25–28.

————. (1998). How to assess critical thinking in clinical practice. *Dimensions of Critical Care Nursing, 17,* 322–327.

Oermann, M. H., & Gaberson, K. (1998). *Evaluation and testing in nursing education.* New York: Springer.

Overholser, J. C. (1992). Socrates in the classroom. *College Teaching, 40*(1), 14–19.

Paul, R. W. (1993). *Critical thinking: How to prepare students for a rapidly changing world.* Santa Rosa, CA: Foundation for Critical Thinking.

Reilly, D. E., & Oermann, M. H. (1992). *Clinical teaching in nursing education* (2nd ed.). New York: National League for Nursing.

Schell, K. (1998). Promoting student questioning. *Nurse Educator, 23*(5), 8–12.

Stokes, L. (1998). Teaching in the clinical setting. In D. M. Billings & J. A. Halstead, *Teaching in nursing* (pp. 281–297). Philadelphia: Saunders.

Wang, A. M., & Blumberg, P. (1983). A study on interaction techniques of nursing faculty in the clinical area. *Journal of Nursing Education, 22,* 144–150.

Wink, D. M. (1993). Using questioning as a teaching strategy. *Nurse Educator, 18*(5), 11–15.

————. (1995). The effective clinical conference. *Nursing Outlook, 43,* 29–32.

13

Written Assignments

Written assignments enable students to develop problem-solving and critical thinking skills, learn about concepts and theories for clinical practice, examine values and beliefs that may affect patient care, and at the same time improve writing skills. Written assignments about clinical practice combined with feedback from the teacher provide an effective means of developing students' writing abilities. While writing assignments may vary with each clinical course, depending on the clinical objectives, assignments may be carefully sequenced across courses for students to develop their writing skills as they progress through the nursing program. The teacher is responsible for choosing written assignments that support the learning outcomes of the course.

PURPOSES OF WRITTEN ASSIGNMENTS

Written assignments for clinical learning have four main purposes: (1) assist students in understanding concepts and theories that relate to care of their patients; (2) improve problem-solving and critical thinking skills; (3) examine their own feelings, beliefs, and values generated from their clinical learning experiences; and (4) develop writing skills.

In choosing written assignments for clinical courses, the teacher should first consider the objectives to be met through the assignments. Writing assignments should build on one another to progressively develop students' skills. Another consideration is the number of assignments to be completed. How many assignments are needed to demonstrate mastery? It may be that one assignment well done is sufficient for meeting the clinical objectives, and students may then progress to other learning activities. Teachers should avoid using the same written assignments repeatedly throughout a clinical course rather than choosing assignments for specific learning outcomes.

Promote Understanding of Concepts and Theories

In written assignments students can describe concepts and theories relevant to the care of their patients and can explain how these concepts and theories guide their clinical decisions. Assignments for this purpose need a clear focus to avoid students' merely summarizing and reporting what they read. Shorter assignments that direct students to apply particular concepts and theories to clinical practice may be of greater value in achieving this purpose than longer assignments for which students may summarize readings they completed without any analysis of the meaning of those readings for their particular patients. For instance, students may be asked to select an intervention for a patient with chronic pain and in one page provide a rationale for its use; read a research article related to care of one of their patients, critique the article, and report on their critique and on why the research is or is not applicable to the patient's care; or select a family theory and complete an assessment of a family using this theory.

Improve Problem Solving and Critical Thinking

Written assignments provide an opportunity for students to analyze patient and other problems they have faced in clinical practice, critique their interventions, and propose new approaches. In writing assignments students may analyze data and clinical situations, identify additional assessment data needed for decision making, identify problems, propose alternate solutions, compare interventions, and evaluate the effectiveness of care. Students may be asked to identify assumptions they made about their patients' responses that influenced their clinical decisions, to critique arguments, to take a stand about an issue and develop a rationale to support it, and to draw generalizations about patient care from different clinical experiences.

Assignments geared to critical thinking should give students freedom to develop their ideas and consider alternate perspectives to the problem. If the assignment is too restrictive, students are inhibited in their thinking and ways of approaching the problem.

Written assignments for critical thinking should be short, ranging from one to two paragraphs to a few pages, and should be focused. In developing these assignments, the teacher should avoid activities in which students merely report on the ideas of others. Instead, the assignment should ask students to consider an alternate point of view or a different way of approaching an issue. Short assignments also provide an opportunity for faculty to give prompt feedback to students.

In addition to being short, the assignment should be focused, and directions to students should be clear and unambiguous (Meyers, 1986). For example, students may be asked to prepare a one-page paper comparing the physiological processes of asthma and bronchitis. Rather than writing on everything they read about asthma and bronchitis, students focus their papers on the physiology of these two conditions.

Examples of written assignments for problem solving and critical thinking follow:

- Compare data collected from two patients for whom you have recently cared. What are similarities and differences?
- Describe in one paragraph significant cues in the data you collected from your patient.
- Select one nursing diagnosis you identified for your patient and provide a rationale for it. What is one alternate diagnosis you might also consider and why? Complete this assignment in two typed pages.
- In one page, identify a patient for whom you have cared in this clinical course. Propose one alternate intervention and provide a rationale for its use.
- Compare, in no more than three pages, two interventions appropriate for your patient in terms of their rationale, research base, and effectiveness.
- Analyze an issue you faced in clinical practice, an alternate course of action that you could have used, and why this alternate action would be effective (one-page paper).
- Identify an issue affecting your patient, family, or community. Analyze that issue from two different points of view. Provide a rationale for actions to be taken from both perspectives. How would you approach this issue and why?
- In no more than two paragraphs, list a decision you made today in your clinical practice and provide a rationale and evidence to support that decision.

Examine Feelings, Beliefs, and Values

Written assignments help learners examine feelings generated from caring for patients and reflect on their beliefs and values that might influence that care. Journals, for instance, provide a way for students to record their feelings about a patient or clinical activity and later reflect on these feelings. Assignments may be developed for students to identify their own beliefs and values and analyze how they affect their interactions with clients. Value-based statements may be given to students for written critique, or students may be asked to analyze an ethical issue, propose alternate courses of actions, and take a stand on the issue.

Develop Writing Skills

An important outcome of writing assignments is the development of skill in communicating ideas in written form. Assignments help students learn how to organize thoughts and present them clearly. The key characteristic of effective writing is the ability to present ideas clearly (Day, 1998). This clarity in writing about clinical practice and care of patients develops through planned writing activities integrated in the nursing program. As a skill, writing ability requires practice, and students need to complete planned writing assignments across clinical courses. All too often, writing assignments are not sequenced progressively across courses or levels in the program; students, then, do not have the benefit of building writing skills sequentially.

Writing-to-learn programs are designed to meet this need. In these programs, written assignments are sequenced across the nursing curriculum. McCarthy and Bowers (1994) described a program in which early courses in the curriculum require short, focused papers in which students summarize, in a few sentences, key points from kectures and readings. Subsequent written assignments of varying lengths are integrated in other courses in the nursing program. Broussard and Oberleitner (1997) have students write brief newspaper columns about clinical topics of interest to consumers; in the senior year students, in collaboration with a faculty mentor, prepare manuscripts with a clinical focus for publication.

A benefit of this planned approach to teaching writing is faculty feedback, provided through drafts and rewrites of papers. A common feature of writing assignments is submitting drafts for feedback. Drafts are essential to foster development of writing skill. They should be critiqued by faculty members for accuracy of content, development of ideas, organization, clarity of expression, and writing skills such as sentence structure, punctuation, and spelling. Sigsby (1992) added that faculty not only should give feedback on writing style but also should teach students how to use a style manual and cite references in their written work.

Small group critique of each other's writing also is appropriate, particularly for formative purposes. This small group critique provides a basis for subsequent revisions and gives feedback to students about both content and writing style. While students may not identify every error in sentence structure and punctuation, they can provide valuable feedback on content, organization, how the ideas are developed, and clarity of writing. If the assignment will be graded at a later point, students may use the grading criteria as a guideline for their peer review.

TYPES OF WRITING ASSIGNMENTS
FOR CLINICAL LEARNING

There are many types of writing assignments appropriate for enhancing clinical learning. Some of these assignments help students better understand the content they are writing about but do not necessarily improve writing skill, whereas other assignments also promote competency in writing. For example, structured assignments such as care plans provide minimal opportunity for freedom of expression, originality, and creativity. Other assignments, though, such as term papers on clinical topics, promote understanding of new content and its use in clinical practice as well as writing ability. The importance of learning how to write clearly should not be underestimated. Poor writing style may prevent a nurse from sharing a great idea (Barnum, 1995).

Types of written assignments for clinical learning include nursing care plan, concept map, concept analysis paper, case method and study, teaching plan, interaction analysis, journal, group writing, free writing, and portfolio.

Nursing Care Plan

Nursing care plans enable students to analyze patients' health problems and design plans of care. The format of the care plan may be developed by the teacher for the clinical course or may be the one used in the clinical agency. In many settings the plan of care is computerized and may be interdisciplinary. Students should move quickly into use of the agency's care plan regardless of its format.

While many teachers espouse the use of nursing care plans for clinical learning, concerns may be raised about the number of care plans students complete in a clinical course and whether or not they actually promote achievement of the learning objectives. Completing a written care plan may help the student identify nursing and other interventions for specific problems, but whether or not that same care plan promotes problem-solving learning and critical thinking is questionable. Often students develop their care plans from the literature or ones already completed in the clinical setting without thinking about the content themselves. Even if the care plan is the most appropriate written assignment for the objectives, the question still remains as to how many care plans students need to complete in a clinical course to meet these objectives.

Concept Map

A concept or cognitive map is a graphic or pictorial arrangement of key concepts that relate to a patient's care. Concept maps present a hierarchical structure of concepts that help students connect new information and retain knowledge more effectively over time (All & Havens, 1997). Mapping concepts visually helps students connect key ideas together in a meaningful way. A concept map acts as a road map for students, showing important concepts related to patient care and the pathways that connect them. Beitz (1998) described a concept map as a two-dimensional schematic device composed of concepts and linking words or symbols arranged in a hierarchy.

There are many uses of concept maps in clinical learning. First, students may complete a concept map from their readings to assist them in linking new facts and concepts to their own patients. The readings students complete for clinical practice, and in nursing courses overall, contain vast amounts of facts and specific information; concept maps help students process this information in a meaningful way, linking new and existing ideas together. Second, concept maps are useful in student preparation for clinical practice (All & Havens, 1997; Kathol, Geiger, & Hartig, 1998). Concept maps may be completed prior to a patient care assignment to assist students in organizing data and planning the patient's care. Third, concept maps may be developed collaboratively by students in clinical conferences. For this purpose, students may present a patient for whom they have cared, with the clinical group then developing a concept map about that patient's care. Alternately, the clinical group may develop a concept map about conditions or community problems they are learning about in the course. Students may be asked to illustrate their work on a poster board. Small group development of concept maps enhances critical thinking, learning from one another, and group process; it also allows for feedback from the teacher.

Concept maps are organized with more specific concepts written under more general ones. Students first identify relevant concepts for their patients' care, then they link these concepts together. Figure 13.1 is an example of a concept map. All and Havens (1997) suggested that two or three versions of the map may be needed for meaningful learning to occur. The teacher's role is to provide feedback and allow for flexibility in how students develop their maps. Individual variation should be expected in the structure and appearance of each student's cognitive map (Irvine, 1995).

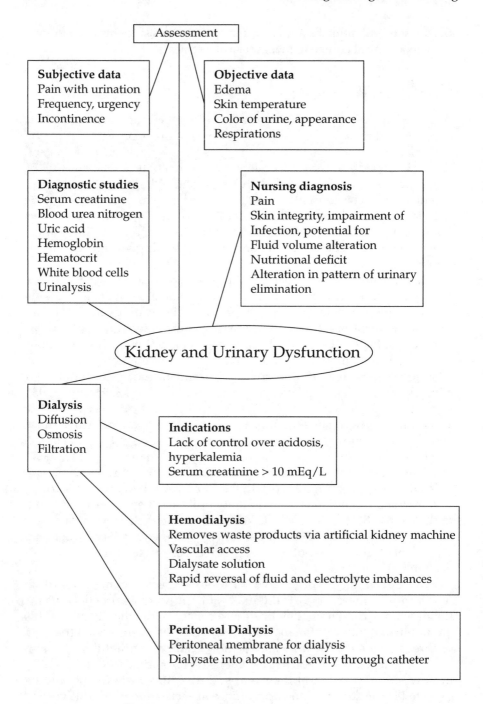

Figure 13.1 Example of a concept map.

Baugh and Mellott (1998) described a four-step process for developing concept maps: (1) diagram pertinent conditions, such as COPD (Chronic Obstructive Pulmonary Disease), renal insufficiency, and congestive heart failure; (2) cluster data and clinical manifestations with the appropriate concepts, such as increased potassium, creatinine, and BUN (blood urea nitrogen) with renal insufficiency; (3) cluster data and therapeutics with the appropriate concepts, such as digoxin with congestive heart failure; (4) link the concepts by arrows, direct lines, or broken lines, indicating the nature of the relationship.

Concept Analysis Paper

Concept analysis papers, on concepts related to clinical practice, help students understand difficult concepts and how they are used in patient care. For these papers, students identify and define the concept, such as chronic pain; examine characteristics and attributes of the concept; develop or present clinical cases that reflect the concept, related nursing interventions, and a rationale as to their effectiveness; and describe how the concept is operationalized in these cases and other similar clinical situations (Swansburg, 1995).

Case Method and Case Study

Case method and case study describe a clinical situation, developed around an actual or hypothetical patient, for student review and critique. In case method the case provided for analysis is generally shorter and more specific than in case study. Case studies are more comprehensive in nature, thereby presenting a complete picture of the patient and clinical situation. After analyzing the case, students complete written questions about it; questions may be answered individually or by small groups of students. Case method and case study are discussed in detail in Chapter 11.

Teaching Plan

Teaching plans enable students to apply concepts of learning and teaching to patients, families, and communities. This is another type of written assignment that may be completed individually or in small groups. After developing the teaching plan, students may use it as a basis for their teaching. There are many formats for teaching plans, but typically the assignment would include: objectives, content, teaching strategies, and evaluation strategies.

Interaction Analysis

Interaction analysis, or process recording, provides a means for students to record and then analyze their interactions with patients, families, staff, and others in the clinical setting. Depending on the objectives to be met, students may analyze verbal and nonverbal behaviors of participants in the interaction; their feelings, beliefs, and values and how these might have influenced the interaction; the specific communication skills they used and their effectiveness; and strengths and weaknesses of the interaction.

Journal

Journal writing assists students in relating theory to clinical practice and linking their readings and classroom instruction to care of patients. Journals may further students' critical thinking (Callister, 1993; Sedlak, 1992, 1997).

Writing in journals about clinical practice provides opportunities for students to

- reflect on their clinical learning activities
- document feelings generated from their clinical practice
- "think aloud" and record their perceptions of their clinical learning activities (Brown & Sorrell, 1993)
- disclose student perceptions that help the teacher better understand student behavior (Mann, 1996)
- record accomplishments and what they learned in clinical practice
- develop self-esteem (Heinrich, 1992)
- communicate with the teacher.

Journals are not as effective as other assignments for developing writing skills, but they provide an avenue for expressing feelings and dialoguing with the teacher about them.

Hodges (1996) proposed leveling journal writing through a curriculum to promote progressive development of cognitive skills. In this model, students begin with journal entries that require summarization of clinical learning activities and descriptions of responses to their clinical experiences; later, they analyze and critique different positions, issues, and views of others.

There are different ways of structuring journals, and the decision should rest with the intended outcomes of using the journal in the clinical course. Brown and Sorell (1993) recommended that the teacher first specify the learning outcomes and goals to be met through journal writing, such as documenting observations of patients, then describe how journal entries should be made. Thoughtful and prompt feedback from the teacher is required to develop a dialogue with the student.

Another set of guidelines for clinical journal writing is more specific. In this model (Patton et al., 1997), students write a journal entry on a significant clinical incident. The incident represents a "patient care episode that stimulated their thinking" (p. 238). For each journal entry, students discuss five of the following areas:

1. Nursing interventions they or others carried out in the clinical setting
2. Their decision-making process
3. What they would do differently when a similar incident occurs
4. Their analysis of the clinical incident
5. Previously learned knowledge and clinical experiences that helped them with the current clinical situation
6. Description of their competency
7. Their areas of strengths and weaknesses and their feelings, thoughts, and perceptions
8. Resources they used with a rationale (Patton et al., 1997, p. 238).

Journals typically are not graded but provide an opportunity for giving feedback to learners. Students have greater freedom in recording feelings, ideas, and responses when the journal is not graded and is used only for giving feedback to them. Hodges (1996), however, proposed that journals could be evaluated and graded on grammar, spelling, sentence structure, clarity, logical flow of argument, and substantive critical thought (p. 140). Most experts, though, do not recommend grading journals. Assigning a grade can suppress the "introspection, reflection, and dialogue that facilitate exploration and articulation of clinical nursing" (Holmes, 1997, p. 491).

Group Writing

Not all writing assignments need to be done by students individually. There is much to be gained with group writing exercises as long as the groups are small and the exercises are carefully focused. Short written assignments, such as analyzing an issue and reporting in writing the outcomes of the analysis or developing a care plan or teaching protocol as a group, may be completed in clinical conferences. These group assignments provide experience for students in expressing their ideas to others in the group and working collaboratively in communicating the results of their thinking as a group in written form.

Free Writing

Free writing is continuous and rapid writing, with the goal of getting ideas onto paper without consideration of format and grammar (Bradley-Springer, 1993). Students may be given a short time, for instance, 10 minutes in a clinical conference, to write about their feelings generated from the clinical learning activities they completed, the patient for whom they cared, or their community experiences. Or they may be asked to identify an issue they faced in their clinical practice and how they felt about that issue.

Free writing also may be done prior to clinical learning activities to determine what students have learned from their readings and to identify questions and gaps in their learning. Free writing assignments help students transfer learning from the class to their clinical practice (Jensen, 1994). For free writing assignments, only a short period of time should be allowed, since the purpose is to get ideas on paper without concern about writing style. Students may then discuss their ideas with their peers.

Portfolio

A portfolio provides an opportunity for students to present projects they completed in their clinical courses over a period of time. Portfolios are collections of projects students developed and worked on for significant periods of time that demonstrate their learning (Bott, 1996, p. 190). They may include evidence of student learning for a series of clinical experiences, over the duration of a clinical course, or for documenting competencies in terms of curriculum or program outcomes (Oermann & Gaberson, 1998).

There are two types of portfolios: best-work and growth and learning progress (Nitko, 1996). Best-work portfolios include materials and products developed by students in clinical practice that demonstrate their learning and achievements. These portfolios reflect the best work of the students in the clinical course. In contrast, growth and learning progress portfolios include materials and products in the process of being developed. These portfolios serve as a way of monitoring students' progress in clinical practice (Oermann & Gaberson, 1998). With both types of portfolios, the teacher reviews them periodically and provides feedback on the materials and products in the portfolio.

The content of the portfolio depends on the clinical objectives to be achieved. Students may include in their portfolios any materials they developed individually or in a group that provide evidence of their achieving the clinical objectives. Examples of materials are:

- nursing care plans
- teaching plans
- short papers written about clinical practice
- concept maps
- cases analyzed individually or by the clinical group
- other writing assignments completed in the clinical course
- their journal or entries similar to those put in a journal
- interaction analyses
- reports of group work
- reports and observations made in the clinical setting
- a self-assessment
- reflections of their patient care experiences and meaning to them
- other products completed in clinical practice.

Table 13.1 presents a process for developing a portfolio for a clinical course.

EVALUATING WRITTEN ASSIGNMENTS

Written assignments may be evaluated formatively or summatively. Formative evaluation provides feedback to students for their continued learning but not for grading purposes. Periodic assessment of drafts of papers and work in progress is formative in nature and is not intended for arriving at a grade. Summative evaluation of completed writing assignments is designed for grading the assignment, not for giving feedback to the student.

For written assignments that are not graded, the teacher's role is to give prompt and sufficient feedback for students to learn from the assignment. If the assignment will be graded at a later time, however, then criteria for grading should be established and communicated to the learner. Any assignment that will eventually be graded should have clear, specific, and measurable criteria for evaluation. Some writing assignments, such as journals, do not lend themselves to grading and instead are best used for formative evaluation only.

Drafts

If drafts of written assignments are to be submitted, the teacher should inform students of each required due date. All written assignments benefit from prompt and specific feedback from the teacher. Feedback should be given on the quality of the content, as reflected in the criteria for evaluation, and on writing style, if appropriate for the assignment. Students

Table 13.1 Developing a Portfolio for Clinical Learning

Step 1: Identify the purposes of the portfolio.

- Will the portfolio serve as a means of monitoring students' development of clinical competencies, focusing predominantly on the growth of students? Will the portfolio provide evidence of students' best work in clinical practice, including products reflecting their learning over a period of time? Or, will the portfolio meet both demands, enabling the teacher to give continual feedback to students on the process of learning and projects on which they are working as well as providing evidence of their accomplishments and achievements in clinical practice?

- Will the portfolio be used for formative or summative evaluation? Both?

- Will the portfolio be developed for a series of clinical learning activities, over the length of a clinical course, or over the length of the curriculum?

- Will the portfolio serve as a means of assessing prior learning and therefore have an impact on the types of learning activities or courses that students complete, for instance, for assessing the prior learning of RNs entering a baccalaureate or higher degree program or for licensed practical nurses entering an associate degree program?

- What is the student's role in defining the focus and content of the portfolio?

Step 2: Identify the type of entries and content to be included in the portfolio.

- What types of entries are required in the portfolio, for example, products developed by students, descriptions of projects with which students are involved, descriptions of clinical learning activities and reactions to them, observations made in clinical practice and analysis of them, and papers completed by students?

- In addition to required entries, what other types of content and entries might be included in the portfolio?

- Who determines the content of the portfolio and types of entries? Teacher only? Student only? Both?

- Will the entries be the same for all students or individualized by the student?

- What is the minimum number of entries?

- How should the entries in the portfolio be organized, or will students organize it themselves?

Table 13.1 *(continued)*

- What is the time frame for each entry to be included in the portfolio, and at what points in time should it be submitted to faculty for review and feedback?
- Will teacher and student meet in a conference for discussion of the portfolio?

Step 3: Decide on the evaluation of the portfolio entries, including criteria for evaluation of individual entries and the portfolio overall.

- How will the portfolio be integrated within the clinical evaluation grade and course grade, if at all?
- What criteria will be used to evaluate, and perhaps score, each type of entry and the portfolio as a whole?
- Will only the teacher evaluate the portfolio and its entries? Or will students evaluate their own progress and work? Or will the evaluation be a collaborative effort?

Adapted from *Evaluation and Testing in Nursing Education* (pp. 194–195), by M. H. Oermann and K. B. Gaberson, 1998. New York: Springer. Copyright 1998 by Springer. Adapted with permission.

need specific suggestions about revisions, not general statements such as "Unclear objectives in teaching plan." Instead, tell students exactly what needs to be changed, for instance, "Objective #1 in teaching plan is not measurable. Revise the verb; content is clear and relevant." Drafts of written assignments are important because they serve as a means of improving writing and thinking about the content. Prompt, clear, and specific feedback about revisions is essential to meet this purpose. Drafts in most instances are used for feedback and therefore are not graded.

Criteria for Evaluation

The criteria for evaluation should relate to the learning objectives to be met with the assignment. For example, if students write a short paper to meet the objective "Compare interventions for nausea associated with chemotherapy," the criteria should relate to the appropriateness of the interventions selected for critique, how effectively the student compared them, the rationale developed for the analysis, and the like.

General criteria for evaluating written assignments follow. These criteria need to be adapted based on the type of assignment and its intent. For assignments that are graded, students should have the criteria for evaluation and scoring protocol at the time the assignment is made so they can develop it with these criteria in mind.

1. *Content*
   Content is relevant.
   Content is accurate.
   Significant concepts and theories are presented.
   Concepts and theories are applied to clinical situation and used for the analysis.
   Content is comprehensive.
   Content reflects current research.
   Hypotheses, conclusions, and decisions are supported.
   Content is individualized to patient, family, and community

2. *Organization*
   Content is organized logically.
   Ideas are presented in a logical sequence.
   Ideas are described clearly.

3. *Process*
   Process used to arrive at solutions, approaches, decisions, and so forth is adequate.
   Consequences of decisions are considered and weighed.
   A sound rationale is provided.
   For papers on analysis of issues, the rationale supports the position taken.
   Multiple perspectives and new approaches are considered.

4. *Writing Style*
   Sentence structure is clear.
   There are no grammatical errors.
   There are no spelling errors.
   Appropriate punctuation is used.
   The length of the paper is consistent with requirements.
   References are cited appropriately throughout the paper.
   References are cited accurately according to the required format.

Grading Assignments

In grading written assignments, a scoring protocol should be developed based on the criteria established for evaluation. The scoring protocol must be used in the same way for all students. This is an important principle in grading written assignments to ensure consistency across papers. Also, some teachers tend to be more lenient, and others tend to be more critical in their review of papers. A scoring protocol helps the teacher base the grade on the established criteria rather than on some other standard. Teachers will be more consistent in grading papers if they first establish specific criteria for evaluation, then develop a scoring protocol based on these criteria, and lastly use that scoring protocol in the same way for each student.

This also is important because sometimes the student's writing ability influences, either positively or negatively, the evaluation of the paper overall. In grading written assignments, keep the criteria separate; evaluate content, organization, process, and writing style based on the specific criteria for each area without having the scores in one area influence the others.

Written assignments that are graded should be read anonymously if at all possible. This is sometimes difficult with small groups of students. Nevertheless, ask students to record their student numbers on their papers rather than their names. There is a tendency in evaluating papers and other written assignments, similar to essay items, for the teacher to be influenced by a general impression of the student. This is called the halo effect. The teacher may have positive or negative feelings about the student or other biases that may influence evaluating and grading the assignment.

Another reason to read papers anonymously is to avoid a "carryover effect." In this situation the teacher carries an impression of the quality of one written assignment to the next one that the student completes. If the student develops an outstanding paper, the teacher may be influenced to score subsequent written assignments at a similarly high level; the same situation may occur with a poor paper. The teacher therefore "carries" the impression of the student from one written assignment to the next. If there are multiple questions that students answered as part of a written assignment, cover up previous scores so as not to be biased about the quality of the next answer. Evaluate all students' answers to one question before proceeding to the next question (Oermann & Gaberson, 1998).

All written assignments should be read twice before scoring. In the first reading, note errors in content, omission of major content areas, problems with organization, problems with the process used for approaching the problem or issue, and problems with writing style. Record comments on the student's paper with suggestions for revision. After reading through all of the papers, begin a second reading for scoring purposes. Reading the papers twice also gives the teacher a sense of how students approached the assignment. In some cases the scoring protocol may need to be revised.

Papers and other types of written assignments should be read in random order. After the first reading, shuffle the papers so they are read in a random order the second time through. Papers read early may be scored higher than those read near the end (Oermann & Gaberson, 1998). Teacher fatigue also may set in and influence grading of the papers. While this section of the chapter dealt with grading written assignments, the teacher should remember that many of these assignments will not be graded.

SUMMARY

Written assignments for clinical learning have four main purposes: (1) assist students in understanding concepts and theories that relate to care of their patients; (2) improve problem-solving and critical thinking skills; (3) examine their own feelings, beliefs, and values generated from their clinical learning experiences; and (4) develop writing skills. Not all writing assignments achieve each of these outcomes. The teacher decides first on the outcomes to be met, then plans the writing assignment with these outcomes in mind.

Written assignments for critical thinking should be short. In developing these assignments, the teacher should avoid activities in which students merely report on the ideas of others. Instead, the assignment should ask students to consider an alternate point of view or a different way of approaching an issue. Short assignments also provide an opportunity for faculty to give prompt feedback to students.

Written assignments help learners examine feelings generated from caring for patients and reflect on their beliefs and values that might influence that care. They also help students learn how to organize thoughts and present them clearly. Some nursing faculty have developed writing-to-learn programs whereby written assignments are sequenced across the nursing curriculum.

Types of written assignments for clinical learning include nursing care plan, concept map, concept analysis paper, case method and study, teaching plan, interaction analysis, journal, group writing, free writing, and portfolio. Each of these types was described in the chapter.

Written assignments may be evaluated formatively or summatively. Formative evaluation provides feedback to students for their continued learning but not for grading purposes. Periodic assessment of drafts of papers and work in progress is formative in nature and is not intended for arriving at a grade. Summative evaluation of completed writing assignments is designed for grading the assignment, not for giving feedback to the student.

In grading written assignments, a scoring protocol should be developed based on the criteria established for evaluation. The scoring protocol must be used in the same way for all students. Many written assignments, though, are not graded.

REFERENCES

All, A. C., & Havens, R. L. (1997). Cognitive/concept mapping: A teaching strategy for nursing. *Journal of Advanced Nursing, 25*, 1210–1219.

Barnum, B. S. (1995). *Writing and getting published.* New York: Springer.

Baugh, N. G., & Mellott, K. G. (1998). Clinical concept mapping as preparation for student nurses' clinical experiences. *Journal of Nursing Education, 37*, 253–256.

Beitz, J. M. (1998). Concept mapping: Navigating the learning process. *Nurse Educator, 23*(5), 35–41.

Bott, P. A. (1996). *Testing and assessment in occupational and technical education.* Boston: Allyn & Bacon.

Bradley-Springer, L. (1993). Discovery of meaning through imagined experience, writing, and evaluation. *Nurse Educator, 18*(5), 5, 7–10.

Broussard, P. C., & Oberleitner, M. G. (1997). Writing and thinking: A process to critical understanding. *Journal of Nursing Education, 36*, 334–336.

Brown, H. N., & Sorrell, J. M. (1993). Use of clinical journals to enhance critical thinking. *Nurse Educator, 18*(5), 16–19.

Callister, L. C. (1993). The use of student journals in nursing education: Making meaning out of clinical experience. *Journal of Nursing Education, 32*, 185–186.

Day, R. A. (1998). *How to write and publish a scientific paper* (5th ed.). Phoenix: Oryx Press.

Heinrich, K. T. (1992). The intimate dialogue: Journal writing by students. *Nurse Educator, 17*(6), 17–21.

Hodges, H. F. (1996). Journal writing as a mode of thinking for RN-BSN students: A leveled approach to learning to listen to self and others. *Journal of Nursing Education, 35*, 137–141.

Holmes, V. (1997). Grading journals in clinical practice: A delicate issue. *Journal of Nursing Education, 36*, 489–492.

Irvine, L. (1995). Can concept mapping be used to promote meaningful learning in nursing education? *Journal of Advanced Nursing, 21*, 1175–1179.

Jensen, M. (1994). Free writing assignments. *Nurse Educator, 19*(5), 27, 39.

Kathol, D. D., Geiger, M. L., & Hartig, J. L. (1998). Clinical correlation map: A tool for linking theory and practice. *Nurse Educator, 23*(4), 31–34.

Mann, S. A. (1996). Respect: Improving student writing. *Nurse Educator, 21*(4), 34–36.

McCarthy, D. O., & Bowers, B. (1994). Implementation of writing-to-learn in a program of nursing. *Nurse Educator, 19*(3), 32–35.

Meyers, C. (1986). *Teaching students to think critically.* San Francisco: Jossey-Bass.

Nitko, A. J. (1996). *Educational assessment of students* (2nd ed.). Englewood Cliffs, NJ: Prentice-Hall.

Oermann, M. H., & Gaberson, K. B. (1998). *Evaluation and testing in nursing education.* New York: Springer.

Patton, J. G., Woods, S. J., Agarenzo, T., Brubaker, C., Metcalf, T., & Sherrer, L. (1997). Enhancing the clinical practicum experience through journal writing. *Journal of Nursing Education, 36*, 238–240.

Sedlak, C. A. (1992). Use of clinical logs by beginning nursing students and faculty to identify learning needs. *Journal of Nursing Education, 33*, 389–394.

————. (1997). Critical thinking of beginning baccalaureate nursing students during the first clinical nursing course. *Journal of Nursing Education, 36,* 11–18.
Sigsby, L. M. (1992). The importance of writing style. *Nurse Educator, 17*(3), 23.
Swansburg, R. C. (1995). Nominal group techniques. In B. Fuszard (Ed.), *Innovative
teaching strategies in nursing* (2nd ed., pp. 93–100). Gaithersburg, MD: Aspen.

14

Using Preceptors as Clinical Teachers

As discussed in Chapter 4, the preceptor teaching model is an alternative to the traditional clinical teaching model. It is based on the assumption that a consistent one-to-one relationship between an experienced nurse and a nursing student or novice staff nurse is an effective way of providing individualized guidance in clinical learning as well as opportunities for professional socialization (Kersbergen & Hrobsky, 1996; Stokes, 1998). Preceptorships have been used extensively with senior nursing students, graduate students preparing for advanced practice roles, and new staff nurse orientees, but they also have been used effectively with beginning nursing students (Kersbergen & Hrobsky, 1996; LeGris & Côte, 1997; Nordgren, Richardson, & Laurella, 1998; Stokes, 1998). This chapter discusses the effective use of preceptors as clinical teachers. The advantages and disadvantages of preceptorships are examined and suggestions are made for selecting, preparing, evaluating, and rewarding preceptors.

PRECEPTORSHIP MODEL OF CLINICAL TEACHING

A preceptorship is a time-limited, one-one-one relationship between a learner and an experienced nurse who is employed by the health care agency in which the learning activities take place. The teacher is not physically present during the learning activities; the preceptor provides intensive, individualized learning opportunities that improve the learner's clinical competence and confidence. Regardless of learners' levels of education and experience, preceptorships provide opportunities for social-ization into professional nursing roles (Davis & Barham, 1989; LeGris & Côte, 1997; Nordgren et al., 1998; Stokes, 1998).

In a preceptorship model, the teacher is a faculty member or educator who has overall responsibility for the quality of the clinical teaching and learning. The teacher provides the link between the educational program and the practice setting by selecting and preparing preceptors, assigning students to preceptors, providing guidance for the selection of appropri-ate learning activities, serving as a resource to the preceptor-student pair, and evaluating student and preceptor performance. The preceptor func-tions as a role model and provides individualized clinical instruction, sup-port, and socialization for the learner (Stokes, 1998). The preceptor also participates in the evaluation of learner performance, although the teacher has ultimate responsibility for summative evaluation decisions.

USE OF PRECEPTORSHIPS IN NURSING EDUCATION

In academic programs that prepare nurses for initial entry into practice, pre-ceptorships usually are used for students in their last semester, but provid-ing preceptors for beginning students may have even greater benefits. Beginning students may gain from the individual attention of the preceptor and from assignments that help them to expand their basic skills, develop independence, and improve their self-confidence (Nordgren et al., 1998).

Preceptorships frequently are used in graduate programs that prepare nurses for advanced clinical practice, administration, and education roles. At this level, a preceptorship involves well-defined learning objectives based on the student's past clinical, administrative, and teaching experi-ence. The student observes and participates in learning activities that demonstrate functional role components, allowing rehearsal of role behav-iors before actually assuming an advanced practice, administrative, or teaching role. The preceptor must be an expert practitioner who can model the role functions of advanced practice nurses, including decision making, leadership, teaching, problem solving, and scholarship (Kimmel, 1989).

In many health care organizations, preceptors participate in the orien-tation of newly hired staff nurses. Preceptors in these settings act as role models for new staff nurses and support them in their transition into pro-fessional practice or socialization into new roles. They work one on one with new staff nurses, but there is wide variation in the scope of the pre-ceptor role. In some settings, the preceptor merely is a more experienced peer who works side by side with the orientee; in other settings, the pre-ceptor role is more formally that of clinical teacher. Successful preceptorship programs for new staff nurses can improve staff retention and recruitment (Bain, 1996; Hill & Lowenstein, 1992).

There are limited research findings regarding the effectiveness of the preceptor teaching model. Some early studies showed no difference in student performance between students assigned to preceptors and those taught in the traditional clinical teaching model. Some investigators presented anecdotal evidence from preceptors, teachers, and students that preceptorships enhanced student performance. Students who are assigned to preceptors usually report satisfaction due to increased confidence and independence (Stokes, 1998). The decision to use preceptors for clinical teaching, therefore, should be based on the perceived benefits to students and the educational program, after a careful evaluation of the potential advantages and disadvantages.

ADVANTAGES AND DISADVANTAGES OF USING PRECEPTORS

The use of preceptors in clinical teaching has both advantages and disadvantages for the involved parties. Effective collaboration is required to minimize the drawbacks and achieve advantages for the educational program, clinical agency, teachers, preceptors, and students (LeGris & Côte, 1997).

Advantages and Disadvantages for Preceptors and Clinical Agencies

Preceptorships hold many potential advantages for preceptors and the clinical agencies that employ them. The presence of students in the clinical environment tends to enhance the professional development, leadership, and teaching skills of preceptors. While preceptors enjoy sharing their clinical knowledge and skill, they also appreciate the stimulation of working with students who challenge the status quo and raise questions about clinical practice. The interest and enthusiasm of students often is rewarding to nurses who take on the additional responsibilities of the preceptor role (LeGris & Côte, 1997). Students may assist preceptors with research or teaching projects. In agencies that use a clinical ladder, serving as a preceptor may be a means of advancing professionally within the system. The preceptorship model also produces opportunities to recruit potential staff members for the agency from among students who work with preceptors.

The greatest drawback of preceptorships to agencies and preceptors usually is the expected time commitment. Some clinical agencies may not agree to provide preceptors because of increased patient acuity and decreased staff levels, or potential preceptors may decline to participate because of the perception that to do so would add to their workloads (LeGris & Côte, 1997; Nordgren et al., 1998).

Advantages and Disadvantages for Students

Students who participate in preceptorships enjoy a number of benefits. They have the advantage of working one on one with experts who can coach them to increased clinical competence and performance. Preceptorships also provide opportunities for students to experience the realities of clinical practice, including scheduling learning activities on evening and night shifts and weekends in order to follow their preceptors' schedules (LeGris & Côte, 1997; Nordgren et al., 1998).

However, following their preceptors' schedules often creates conflicts with students' academic, work, and family commitments. Additionally, a preceptor's patient assignment may not always be appropriate for a student's clinical learning objectives (Nordgren et al., 1998).

Advantages and Disadvantages for the Educational Program

Preceptorships offer many advantages for the educational program in which they are used. The use of preceptors provides more clinical teachers for students and thus more intensive guidance of students' learning activities. Working collaboratively with preceptors also helps faculty members to stay informed about the current realities of practice; up-to-date clinical information benefits ongoing curriculum development (LeGris & Côte, 1997).

Several disadvantages related to the use of preceptors may affect educational programs. Contrary to a common belief, teachers' responsibilities do not decrease when students work with preceptors. Initial selection of preceptors, preparation of preceptors and students, and ongoing collaboration and communication with preceptors and students require as much time as with the traditional clinical teaching model, or more. The preceptorship model requires considerable indirect teaching time for the development of relationships with agencies and preceptors and the evaluation of preceptors and students. When preceptors are used as clinical teachers, faculty members may be responsible for a greater number of students in several clinical agencies and feel uncertain whether students are learning the application of theory and research findings to practice (LeGris & Côte, 1997; Nordgren et al., 1998).

SELECTING PRECEPTORS

The success of preceptorships largely depends on the selection of appropriate preceptors; such selection is one of the teacher's most important responsibilities. Most faculty members consider the educational preparation of the preceptor to be important; most academic programs require the preceptor to have at least the degree for which the student is preparing, although insistence on this level of educational preparation does not guarantee that learners will be exposed only to professional role models (Davis & Barham, 1989; Myrick & Barrett, 1994; Pond, McDonough, & Lambert, 1993).

The desire to teach and a willingness to serve as a preceptor are important qualities of potential preceptors. Nurses who feel obligated to enact this role usually do not make enthusiastic, effective preceptors (Hill & Lowenstein, 1992). Additional attributes of effective preceptors include the following (Bain, 1996; Davis & Barham, 1989; Stokes, 1998):

- *Clinical expertise or proficiency, depending on the level of the learner.* Preceptors should be able to demonstrate expert psychomotor, problem-solving, critical thinking, and decision-making skills in their area of clinical focus. Nursing students and new staff nurses need preceptors who are at least proficient clinicians; graduate students need preceptors who are expert clinicians, administrators, or educators, depending on the goals of the preceptorship.

- *Leadership abilities.* Good preceptors are change agents in the health care organizations in which they are employed. They demonstrate effective communication skills and are trusted and respected by their peers.

- *Teaching skill.* Preceptors must understand and use principles of adult learning. They should be able to communicate ideas effectively to learners and give descriptive positive and negative feedback.

- *Professional role behaviors and attitudes.* Because preceptors act as role models for learners, they must demonstrate behaviors that represent important professional values. They are accountable for their actions and accept responsibility for their decisions. Good preceptors demonstrate maturity and self-confidence; their approach to learners is nonthreatening and nonjudgmental. Flexibility, open-mindedness, and a sense of humor are additional attributes of effective preceptors.

The selection of preceptor and setting also should take into account the learner's interest in a specific clinical specialty as well as the need for the development of particular skills. The teacher may ask nurse managers to recommend potential preceptors, but the selection should be made by the teacher. Teachers should not choose preceptors from newly established units or those with recent high staff turnover (Davis & Barham, 1989).

PREPARING THE PARTICIPANTS

Thorough preparation of preceptors and students for their roles also is key to the success of preceptorships. Teachers are responsible for initial orientation and continuing support of all participants; preparation can be formal or informal.

Preceptors

Preparation of preceptors may begin with a general orientation, possibly for groups of potential preceptors at the selected agency. This orientation may include the following information:

- Benefits and challenges of precepting
- Characteristics of a good preceptor
- Principles of adult learning
- Clinical teaching and evaluation methods
- The preceptor's role in developing and implementing an individualized learning contract
- The academic program curriculum structure, framework, and goals (LeGris & Côte, 1997; Stokes, 1998).

After preceptors have been selected, they need a specific orientation to their responsibilities. This orientation may take the form of a face-to-face or telephone conference with the teacher; written guidelines may be used to supplement the conference. Table 14.1 is an example of written guidelines for preceptors of graduate nursing students. The conference and written guidelines may include information such as the following:

- *The educational level and previous experience of the student.* Graduate students need learning activities that build on their previous learning and experience in order to produce advanced practice outcomes. Beginning students may not have developed the knowledge and skill to participate in all of the preceptor's activities.
- *How to choose specific learning activities based on learning objectives.* The teacher may share samples of learning contracts or lists of learning activities to guide the preceptor's selection of appropriate activities for the student. Kersbergen and Hrobsky (1996) pro-

Table 14.1 Sample Guidelines for a Preceptor of a Graduate Nursing Student

Guidelines for Preceptors—MSN Student Role Practicum

The preceptor is expected to:

- Facilitate the student's entry into the health care organization.
- Provide the student with an orientation to the organization.
- After receiving the student's goals for the practicum, provide suggestions for how these goals can be accomplished.
- Assist the student with identifying a project that is consistent with organizational needs and student's interests, abilities, and learning needs.
- Meet with the student at regular intervals to discuss progress on project and achievement of individual and course objectives.
- Provide the student with regular feedback regarding his/her performance.
- Communicate regularly with the faculty member regarding the student's progress.
- At the end of the preceptorship, provide a written evaluation of the student's performance related to the following:
  - goal achievement
  - clinical knowledge and skill
  - problem-solving and decision-making skills
  - communication and presentation skills
  - interpersonal skills

posed the use of a clinical map guide to planning precepted learning activities. Similar to critical pathways used by case managers in a managed care delivery system, clinical maps are tools that guide preceptors and students to select learning activities that meet identified objectives.

- *Scheduling of clinical learning activities.* A common feature of preceptorships is the scheduling of the student's learning activities according to the preceptor's work schedule. Preceptors should be advised of dates on which students and teachers may not be available because of school holidays, examinations, and other course requirements (Kersbergen & Hrobsky, 1996; LeGris & Côte, 1997; Nordgren et al., 1998).

New preceptors have learning needs much like those of students and new staff nurses; supportive role models and coaching are essential to success. Preceptor programs for newly hired staff nurses may hold regular meetings of preceptors with staff development instructors and nurse managers to review material such as adult learning principles, teaching and evaluation strategies, and conflict resolution (Davis & Barham, 1989; Hill & Lowenstein, 1992).

Students

Learners also need to understand the purposes and process of the preceptorship. They need an orientation to the process of planning individual learning activities, an explanation of teacher and preceptor roles, and a review of unit policies specific to student practice (Davis & Barham, 1989; LeGris & Côte, 1997). At the beginning of the preceptorship, teachers should clarify evaluation responsibilities and expectations, such as dates for learning contract approval, site visits, and conferences with faculty members.

IMPLEMENTATION

Successful implementation of preceptorships depends on a mutual understanding of the roles and responsibilities of the participants. Teacher, student, and preceptor collaborate to plan and implement learning activities that will facilitate the student's goal attainment. Key to these processes is effective communication among the participants.

Roles and Responsibilities of Participants

Preceptors are responsible for patient care in addition to clinical teaching of the student. The preceptor is expected to be a positive role model and a resource person for the student. The clinical teaching responsibilities of the preceptor include creating a positive learning climate, including the student in activities that relate to learning goals, and providing feedback to the student and teacher. Sometimes preceptors experience conflict between the teacher and evaluator roles, especially when precepting new staff members. If the learner is unable to perform according to expectations, the faculty member or staff development instructor must be notified so that a plan for correcting the deficiencies may be established (Hill & Lowenstein, 1992; LeGris & Côte, 1997).

The student is expected to participate actively in planning learning activities. Planning may take the form of a learning contract that specifies individualized objectives and clinical learning activities. Because the teacher is not always present during learning activities, the student must communicate frequently with the teacher; communication may take the form of a reflective journal that is shared with the teacher on a regular basis. The student must notify the teacher immediately of any problems encountered in the implementation of the preceptorship. The student's responsibilities also include self-evaluation and evaluation of the preceptor's teaching effectiveness.

As previously discussed, the teacher is responsible for making preceptor selections, pairing students with preceptors, and orienting preceptors and students. The teacher is an important resource to preceptors and students to assist in problem solving, and teacher availability is particularly important to preceptors (Zerbe & Lachat, 1991). Therefore, the teacher must make arrangements for consultation via telephone, e-mail, or long-range pager. The teacher also arranges individual and group conferences with students and preceptors and visits the clinical sites as needed or requested by any of the participants. If students submit reflective journal entries, the teacher responds to them with feedback that helps students to evaluate their progress. Teachers have responsibility for the final evaluation of learner performance with input from preceptors, and they also evaluate the effectiveness of preceptors with input from students.

Planning and Implementing Learning Activities

A common strategy for planning and implementing students' learning activities in the preceptorship model of clinical teaching is the use of an individualized learning contract. A learning contract is an explicit agreement between teacher and student that clarifies expectations of each participant in the teaching-learning process. It specifies the learning goals that have been established, the learning activities selected to meet the objectives, and the expected outcomes and criteria by which they will be evaluated. In a preceptorship, the learning contract is negotiated among teacher, student, and preceptor and serves as a guide for planning and implementing the student's learning activities. Table 14.2 is an example of a learning contract format that could be adapted for any level of learner.

As discussed above, effective communication among the preceptor, student, and teacher is critical to the success of the preceptorship. Communication between teacher and student may be facilitated by the student's keeping a reflective journal and sharing it with the teacher on a regular basis. In the journal, the student describes and analyzes learning activities that relate to the objective, reflecting on the meaning and value of the experiences. The journal entries may be recorded on paper, computer file, or audiotape; the teacher responds with feedback via written comment, e-mail, or audiotaped comment. Additionally, the student and

Table 14.2 Sample Learning Contract Format

Learning Contract

Student Information

Name and credentials:
Address:
Phone number:
Fax number:
E-mail address:

Teacher Information
Name and credentials:
Address:
Phone number:
Fax number:
E-mail address:

Preceptor Information
Name and credentials:
Address:
Phone number:
Fax number:
E-mail address:

Clinical learning objectives	Learning activities and resources	Evaluation evidence, responsibility, and time frame

Starting date: Completion date:

Student Signature   _____   Date _____
Preceptor Signature _____   Date _____
Teacher Signature   _____   Date _____

teacher should have telephone, e-mail, or face-to-face contact as necessary for the teacher to give consultation and guidance. Similarly, the teacher and preceptor should have regular contact by telephone, e-mail, or face-to-face meetings so that the teacher receives feedback about learner performance and offers guidance and consultation as needed.

The realities of clinical and academic cultures present challenges to effective communication among teacher, preceptor, and student. Preceptors often work a variety of shifts, students often have complicated academic and work schedules, and teachers have an assortment of responsibilities in addition to clinical teaching. Flexibility and commitment to establishing and maintaining communication are essential to overcome these challenges (LeGris & Côte, 1997).

EVALUATING THE OUTCOMES

Students, teachers, and preceptors share responsibility for monitoring the progress of learning and for evaluating outcomes of the preceptorship (LeGris & Côte, 1997). Student performance may be evaluated according to the terms specified in the learning contract or through the clinical evaluation methods used by the educational program. If a learning contract is used, student self-evaluation usually is an important strategy for assessing outcomes. As discussed earlier, preceptors are expected to give feedback to the learner and to the teacher, but the teacher has the responsibility for the summative evaluation of learner performance.

An important aspect of evaluation concerns the teaching effectiveness of preceptors. Students are an important source of information about the quality of their preceptors' clinical teaching, but the teacher also should assess the degree to which preceptors were able to effectively guide the students' learning. A modified form of the teaching effectiveness tool used to evaluate clinical teachers may be used to collect data from students regarding their preceptors (Nordgren et al., 1998). Table 14.3 is an example of a form for student evaluation of preceptor teaching effectiveness. Because each preceptor typically is assigned to only one student at a time, it usually is impossible to maintain anonymity of student evaluations. Therefore, teachers may wish to share a summary of the student's evaluation, instead of the raw data, with the preceptor.

REWARDING PRECEPTORS

Preceptors make valuable contributions to nursing education programs, and they should receive appropriate rewards and incentives for their par-

Table 14.3 Sample Tool for Student Evaluation of Preceptor Teaching Effectiveness

---

Student Evaluation of Preceptor's Teaching Effectiveness

Directions: Rate the extent to which each statement describes your preceptor's teaching behaviors by circling a number following each item, using the following scale:

4 = To a large extent
3 = To a moderate extent
2 = To a small extent
1 = Not at all

1. The preceptor was an excellent professional role model.	4 3 2 1
2. The preceptor guided my clinical problem solving.	4 3 2 1
3. The preceptor helped me to apply theory to clinical practice.	4 3 2 1
4. The preceptor was responsive to my individual learning needs.	4 3 2 1
5. The preceptor provided constructive feedback about my performance.	4 3 2 1
6. The preceptor communicated clearly and effectively.	4 3 2 1
7. The preceptor encouraged my independence.	4 3 2 1
8. The preceptor was flexible and open-minded.	4 3 2 1
9. Overall, the preceptor was an excellent clinical teacher.	4 3 2 1
10. I would recommend this preceptor for other students.	4 3 2 1

---

ticipation. At minimum, every preceptor should receive an individualized thank-you letter, specifying some of the benefits that the student received from the preceptorship. A copy of the letter may be sent to the preceptor's supervisor or manager to be used as evidence of clinical excellence at the time of the preceptor's next performance evaluation.

Other formal and informal ways of acknowledging the contributions of preceptors include:

- A name badge that identifies the nurse as a preceptor
- A certificate of appreciation, signed by the administrator of the education program
- An annual preceptor recognition event, including refreshments and an inspirational speaker
- Free or reduced-price registration for continuing education programs

- Reduced-rate tuition for academic courses
- Bookstore gift certificates
- Adjunct or affiliate faculty appointment
- Differential pay or adjustment of work schedule for preceptors who work with new staff members
- A gift, such as a fruit basket or plant (Bain, 1996; LeGris & Côte, 1997).

SUMMARY

The use of preceptors is an alternative to the traditional clinical teaching model based on the assumption that a consistent one-to-one relationship between an experienced nurse and a nursing student or novice staff nurse is an effective way of providing individualized guidance in clinical learning and professional socialization. Preceptorships have been used extensively with senior nursing students, graduate students preparing for advanced practice roles, and new staff nurse orientees.

A preceptorship is a time-limited, one-on-one relationship between a learner and an experienced nurse. The teacher is not physically present during the learning activities; the preceptor provides intensive, individualized learning opportunities that improve the learner's clinical competence and confidence. The teacher has overall responsibility for the quality of the clinical teaching and learning and provides the link between the educational program and the practice setting. The preceptor functions as a role model and provides individualized clinical instruction, support, and socialization for the learner.

Preceptorships frequently are used for students in their last semester of academic preparation for entry into practice and for graduate students preparing for advanced clinical practice, administration, and education roles. In many health care organizations, preceptors participate in the orientation of newly hired staff nurses by acting as role models and supporting new staff members' professional socialization.

The use of preceptors in clinical teaching has both advantages and disadvantages for the educational program, clinical agency, teachers, preceptors, and students. Benefits for preceptors and their employers include the stimulation of working with learners who raise questions about clinical practice, assistance from students with research or teaching projects, rewards through a clinical ladder system for participation as a preceptor, and opportunities to recruit potential staff members for the agency from among students who work with preceptors. The greatest drawback of preceptorships to agencies and preceptors usually is the expected time commitment.

Students experience the benefits of working one on one with clinical experts who can coach them to improve performance as well as opportunities to experience the realities of clinical practice. However, following their preceptors' schedules often creates conflicts with students' academic, work, and family commitments.

Preceptorships offer many advantages to teachers and educational programs. The use of preceptors provides more clinical teachers for students and thus more intensive guidance of students' learning activities. Working collaboratively with preceptors also helps faculty members to stay informed about the current realities of practice. Disadvantages include the amount of indirect teaching time required to select, prepare, and communicate with preceptors and students.

Selection of appropriate preceptors is important to the success of preceptorships. Most academic programs require the preceptor to have at least the degree for which the student is preparing. The desire to teach and a willingness to serve as a preceptor are very important qualities of potential preceptors. Additional attributes of effective preceptors include clinical expertise or proficiency, leadership abilities, teaching skill, and professional role behaviors and attitudes.

Teachers are responsible for initial orientation and continuing support of all participants; preparation can be formal or informal. A general orientation for potential preceptors may include information about benefits and challenges of precepting, characteristics of a good preceptor, principles of adult learning, clinical teaching and evaluation methods, and the structure and goals of the nursing education program. After preceptors have been selected, they need a specific orientation to their responsibilities, including information about the educational level and previous experience of the student, choosing specific learning activities based on learning objectives, and scheduling of clinical learning activities. Learners also need an orientation that includes the purposes of the preceptorship, the process of planning individual learning activities, and an explanation of teacher and preceptor roles.

Successful implementation of preceptorships depends on mutual understanding of the roles and responsibilities of the participants. The preceptor is expected to be a positive role model and a resource person for the student. The responsibilities of the preceptor include creating a positive learning climate, including the student in activities that relate to learning goals, and providing feedback to the student and teacher. The student usually arranges the schedule of clinical learning activities to coincide with the preceptor's work schedule and is expected to participate actively in planning learning activities. Because the teacher is not always present during learning activities, the student must keep the teacher informed about progress through frequent communication. In addition to making preceptor selections and orienting preceptors and students, the teacher is an important resource to preceptors and students to assist in problem solving. Teachers must make adequate arrangements for communication with other participants.

A common strategy for planning and implementing students' learning activities is the use of an individualized learning contract, an explicit agreement among teacher, student, and preceptor that specifies the learning goals, learning activities selected to meet the objectives, and the expected outcomes and criteria by which they will be evaluated. The learning contract serves as a guide for planning and implementing the student's learning activities.

Students, teachers, and preceptors share responsibility for monitoring the progress of learning and for evaluating outcomes of the preceptorship. Student performance is assessed according to the terms specified in the learning contract or through the clinical evaluation methods used by the educational program, through self-evaluation, and through feedback from preceptors. The teacher is responsible the summative evaluation of learner performance. Students are an important source of information about their preceptors' clinical teaching effectiveness, but the teacher also should assess the degree to which preceptors were able to effectively guide students' learning.

Preceptors should receive appropriate rewards and incentives for the contributions they make to the educational program. At minimum, every preceptor should receive an individualized thank-you letter, specifying some of the benefits that the student received from the preceptorship. Other formal and informal ways of acknowledging the contributions of preceptors include name badges, certificates of appreciation, preceptor recognition events, free or reduced-price registration for continuing education programs, reduced-rate tuition for academic courses, bookstore vouchers or similar gifts, adjunct or affiliate faculty appointment, and differential pay.

REFERENCES

Bain, L. (1996). Preceptorship: A review of the literature. *Journal of Advanced Nursing, 24*, 104–107.

Davis, L. L., & Barham, P. D. (1989). Get the most from your preceptorship program. *Nursing Outlook, 37*, 167–171.

Hill, E. M., & Lowenstein, L. E. (1992). Preceptors: Valuable members of the orientation process. *AORN Journal, 55*, 1237–1248.

Kersbergen, A. L., & Hrobsky, P. E. (1996). Use of clinical map guides in precepted clinical experiences. *Nurse Educator, 21*(6), 19–22.

Kimmel, L. H. (1989). Guiding the way: Acting as a preceptor for graduate students. *Journal of Psychosocial Nursing, 27*(11), 14–21.

LeGris, J., & Côte, F. H. (1997). Collaborative partners in nursing education: A preceptorship model for BscN students. *Nursing Connections, 10*(1), 55–70.

Myrick, F., & Barrett, C. (1994). Selecting clinical preceptors for baccalaureate nurs-
    ing students: A critical issue in clinical teaching. *Journal of Advanced Nursing,
    19,* 194–198.
Nordgren, J., Richardson, S. J., & Laurella, V. B. (1998). A collaborative preceptor
    model for clinical teaching of beginning nursing students. *Nurse Educator,
    23*(3), 27–32.
Pond, E., McDonough, J., & Lambert, V. (1993). Preceptors' perceptions of a bac-
    calaureate preceptorial experience. *Nursing Connections, 6,* 15–25.
Reilly, D. E., & Oermann, M. H. (1992). *Clinical teaching in nursing education* (2nd
    ed.). New York: National League for Nursing.
Stokes, L. (1998). Teaching in clinical settings. In D. M. Billings & J. A. Halstead,
    (Eds.), *Teaching in nursing: A guide for faculty* (pp. 281–297). Philadelphia:
    Saunders.
Zerbe, M., & Lachat, M. (1991). A three-tiered team model for undergraduate pre-
    ceptor programs. *Nurse Educator, 16*(2), 18–21.

15

Clinical Teaching in Diverse Settings

Potential practice settings for clinical teaching and learning comprise all places where nurses encounter patients. Acute care hospitals and some community agencies have been the traditional clinical sites for nursing education. However, the goals of clinical teaching and learning may be accomplished in any environment where students can interact with patients: integrated health networks, homes, community centers, schools, workplaces, shelters, hospices, transitional and extended care facilities, day care centers, and the like (Mundt, 1997; Reilly & Oermann, 1992; Stokes, 1998). As the focus of health care becomes more global, wellness-oriented, and population-based, settings for the delivery of care become more diverse, requiring nurse educators to be creative and innovative in using these settings for clinical learning activities. Educating nursing students in such settings also sensitizes them to the needs of diverse populations and enhances recruitment of nursing students to practice in underserved areas to meet current and future staffing needs (LaSala, Hopper, Rissmeyer, & Shipe, 1997; Virgin & Goodrow, 1997). This chapter discusses three trends in clinical teaching: the transition to community care, interdisciplinary clinical education, and the increasing focus on global health care education. It also suggests innovative ways to use traditional and nontraditional settings to meet clinical learning objectives.

TRANSITION TO COMMUNITY-BASED NURSING

Acute care hospitals are becoming less suitable learning environments due to trends in health care delivery that result in declining acute care patient populations and rising acuity levels of patients (Ryan, D'Aoust, Groth, McGee, & Small, 1997). Health care trends make it clear that nursing roles and practice settings will be very different in the future. Patients increasingly are found outside acute care settings, in their homes and communities (Oneha, Magnussen, & Feletti, 1998). Community-based activities help students to learn holistic care of individuals and families in the context of their communities and cultures; practice patient education, including preventive health and self-management; refine their assessment skills; learn to set priorities based on patient needs; identify community health needs and services and resources to meet them; and learn to practice collaboratively with other health care providers (Oneha et al., 1998; Ryan et al., 1997).

For these reasons and others, academic nursing curricula increasingly emphasize community-based nursing. However, "community-based" may be interpreted in two ways: (1) a focus on the care of aggregate populations or community as client or (2) community-based nursing of patients with varying health problems. Most nurses easily can transfer patient care skills from hospital to home settings to meet the needs of patients who were discharged after short inpatient stays. But additional skills such as interpreting epidemiological data, building coalitions to address community problems, assessing community resources, and discerning the impact of environment on health are required for competent care of aggregate populations (Reed & Wuyscik, 1998).

Nursing care in hospitals and community settings is based on different philosophies of practice. In acute care settings, patient care often takes place in specialized units where nursing activities are focused on short-term interventions, patients are relatively dependent, and family access is regulated. In the community, the focus is on the patient within the context of a family and social network. Nursing interventions and goals are defined mutually by nurse and patient, and the purpose of care is to improve function and the quality of life. Despite the differences in philosophy, practice in hospital and community settings does not required widely different knowledge and skills. Nurses in both settings need to plan, organize, coordinate, delegate, provide, and evaluate patient care; identify and mobilize resources; collaborate with other health care providers; and provide for continuity of care (Hunt, 1998).

Teacher and Student Preparation

Successful transition to teaching and learning in community-based settings requires faculty and student preparation. Faculty members who are experienced in acute care of adult patients may have little difficulty transferring their clinical and teaching skills to community-based illness care, but teachers who have little preparation in public health or community practice may require assistance in preparing to teach nursing care of aggregate populations. Teachers may need to develop new clinical skills and revise their teaching methods; faculty development programs and orientation by teachers who have worked in the community may support these adjustments. Faculty preparation for teaching in the community may include reviewing community health textbooks, spending time in the community to become familiar with its characteristics and the population served, and learning the mission, policies, and documentation systems of the agencies that will be used for learning activities (Oneha et al., 1998; Reed & Wuyscik, 1998; Stokes, 1998).

Because students often will be functioning more autonomously in community settings, they need prerequisite interpersonal, problem-solving, and clinical skills. Before entering the community for clinical learning activities, students should practice patient teaching skills, particularly giving anticipatory guidance; solving ill-structured problems that are typical of those encountered in community settings; and analyzing case studies to determine priorities of care (Reed & Wuyscik, 1998). Student preparation for community learning activities also includes special attention to safety precautions. Although it is a common belief that urban areas are more dangerous than suburban, small town, or rural settings, every environment is potentially unsafe to those who do not take necessary precautions. Teachers must provide explicit guidelines for student safety during community learning activities and should document them in the course syllabus. Safety guidelines for home visits should address the following:

- *Communication.* The student should notify the patient of the date and approximate time of the student's visit and verify arrival at the patient's home by a phone call to the agency or the teacher. The student may be asked to carry a cellular phone and should know whom to contact in case of emergency.
- *Travel.* The student should consult a map to plan the route of travel to the patient's home and verify directions with the patient if necessary. If using public transportation, the student needs to know schedules, boarding locations, and fares. If driving to the patient's home, the student needs a well-maintained automobile, sufficient fuel, and possibly coins for parking meters.
- *Dress.* The student must be identifiable as someone who has a legitimate reason for being in the community. Many home care agencies require staff members to wear uniforms, and the student should dress similarly. The student should leave valuables at home or at the agency.
- *Dangerous situations.* The student should leave the setting immediately if there is any doubt as to personal safety. Warning signs of

potential danger include the use of sexual language, drinking or drug-using behavior, the presence of a weapon or a threat to use a weapon, or physical fighting. If the safety of an area is in doubt, the police should be contacted for information (Reed & Wuyscik, 1998).

Meeting the Challenges of Community-based Teaching

The difference in nursing practice between hospital and home environments may require different approaches to teaching. The home environment is more variable, resources are less predictable, access to the patient is not guaranteed and therefore requires planning, and the patient and family members are more autonomous. Teaching in this environment requires indirect guidance of student activities and a more collaborative teaching style (Reed & Wuyscik, 1998). Shifting the focus of clinical teaching to the community challenges long-held, implicit assumptions of how nurses must be prepared to practice, such as:

- Traditional inpatient settings are the best sites for learning essential clinical knowledge.
- Acute-care skills are the most important skills to learn.
- A prescribed sequence of specialty clinical rotations is required.
- Faculty must directly oversee student activities to ensure student learning and evaluate skills (Ryan et al., 1997).

Problem-based, inquiry, and self-directed learning strategies are more appropriate for the development of the independence, critical thinking ability, and problem-solving skills necessary for students to function in community settings (Oneha et al., 1998). Faculty members may not be comfortable with the shift from identical clinical activities for all students to individualized activities that allow students to meet objectives in different ways (Ryan et al., 1997). However, the philosophy of clinical teaching that is discussed in Chapter 1 supports the individualization of learning activities as long as the desired outcome is achieved. Faculty members need to become comfortable with instruction that is less teacher-centered and teacher-controlled; the role of the teacher is that of guide, facilitator, and co-learner (Reed & Wuyscik, 1998; Virgin & Goodrow, 1997).

In addition to preparing existing faculty members for community teaching, qualified community agency personnel may be recruited as preceptors, clinical teaching associates, or clinical teaching partners, with or without joint education-service appointments (Mundt, 1997). See Chapter 4 for a description of the preceptor, clinical teaching associate, and clinical teaching partnership models and Chapter 14 for a more complete discussion of the use of preceptors.

The identification of potential community clinical sites usually is not difficult, but a large number and wide geographic distribution of sites present challenges to the scheduling of clinical activities. Flexible course structures are essential to allow students to participate in realistic community-based activities without conflicts with other course schedules (Oneha et al., 1998; Ryan et al., 1997).

INTERDISCIPLINARY CLINICAL EDUCATION

The education of health care professionals is shifting from the traditional discipline-specific educational models to interdisciplinary education for practice on multiprofessional health teams. The health care environment increasingly requires nurses to collaborate with a variety of health care disciplines in planning, delivering, and evaluating patient care, and students must have clinical learning opportunities that resemble these practice realities. Interdisciplinary clinical education allows students of various health care professions to learn through shared experiences in the same settings, learning about the contributions of each discipline to patient care without competition, paternalism, or sexism (Benson, 1997; LaSala et al., 1997; Stokes, 1998). Interdisciplinary education promotes the development of competency and a professional ethic that supports integrated teamwork. To achieve these outcomes, nursing education as well as education for other health professions must change both within and across disciplines (Bellack et al., 1997).

Clinical settings that are models of interdisciplinary practice are excellent sites for clinical teaching in nursing. Examples of successful interdisciplinary practice settings include geriatric care centers, hospices, rehabilitation centers, trauma centers, and intensive care units (Benson, 1997). For example, acute care nurse practitioner students and physician assistant students can learn to appreciate the interdependency of their roles while practicing together in the intensive care unit, respecting and valuing the contributions that each can make while preserving the autonomy of their respective disciplines. In other settings, nursing, medical, physical therapy, and social work students may participate in regular interdisciplinary clinical conferences.

Planning clinical learning activities in interdisciplinary settings ideally should be done by a multidisciplinary team of teachers. Success in planning such activities requires

- Commitment to the goals of interdisciplinary education and to overcoming resistance to change and curricular rigidity
- Role clarity

- Respect for others' knowledge and skills and appreciation for one another's strengths
- Flexibility and patience in avoiding scheduling conflicts in planning collaborative learning activities
- Clear communication
- The ability to identify philosophical similarities and differences in clinical practice (Bellack et al., 1997; Benson, 1997; Stokes, 1998).

EDUCATION FOR GLOBAL HEALTH CARE

Health problems extend beyond national borders, requiring a global view of health needs and health care. Nursing practice must respond effectively to global health problems related to AIDS and other communicable diseases and to the effects of pollution, malnutrition, substance abuse, and violence (Henry, 1994). Also, since many societies are becoming increasingly diverse, nurses must develop sensitivity to cultural values, beliefs, and traditions in order to provide culturally appropriate care. Cultural variations between patients and nurses may be clinically significant for the diagnosis and treatment of health conditions. If nursing education programs intend to produce graduates who can practice beyond the local area, those graduates must be culturally competent caregivers (Lockhart & Resick, 1997).

Learning activities that take place within the student's own culture and familiar surroundings can fall short of meeting goals for learning cultural competence because the clients' worldviews do not predominate (Kavanagh, 1998). Clinical learning sites in international health settings help students develop cultural sensitivity and competence as well as a global view of nursing and health care (Oneha et al., 1998). Nursing students whose clinical activities take place within other cultures are challenged intellectually and emotionally and must learn to manage culture shock (Kavanagh, 1998).

An example of using international health care settings for clinical learning sites was reported by Ross (1998). A "sister school" collaboration between an American university and a school of nursing at a Nicaraguan university resulted in a number of student and faculty exchange activities focused on community and acute health care. Faculty members from the American university traveled to Nicaragua with groups of baccalaureate, master's, and doctoral students for collaborative learning activities with Nicaraguan nursing students, faculty members, and local health care workers. Students observed health care in local hospitals as well as home and community care in the barrios of Managua and learned to overcome language and cultural barriers in giving nursing care to families. Clinical learning activities in this setting enabled students to meet the objectives of providing holistic care to culturally diverse populations (Ross, 1998).

SELECTING CLINICAL SETTINGS TO SUPPORT CLINICAL TEACHING OBJECTIVES

As discussed in Chapters 3 and 5, the selection of clinical learning activities should be based primarily on the learning objectives. Learning objectives can be achieved in a number of ways and should not prescribe a specific setting where the learning activities must take place. In traditional models of clinical nursing education, students were matched with patients, primarily those hospitalized in acute care facilities, according to their specific health conditions, developmental levels, or acuity of care requirements. However, the growth of managed care systems makes these models of clinical teaching obsolete. Newer health care models are more patient-focused and outcomes-oriented, delivering care in a series of coordinated, multilevel encounters. Students need to learn to assess patient needs and provide and evaluate care across the continuum of care (Mundt, 1997). Creativity and flexibility in considering how objectives might be met will enable clinical teachers to identify a wide variety of clinical settings in which learning activities might occur.

Acute Care Settings

Shorter hospitals stays, lower patient census, and higher acuity levels present challenges to the traditional method of scheduling a group of students to learning activities on a hospital nursing unit. Clinical teachers should consider ways to use nontraditional inpatient settings, such as the operating room, emergency department, and diagnostic procedures units, as learning sites.

The emergency department may be an ideal setting in which students can improve observation skills, practice making triage decisions, and learn to communicate effectively with patients and family members under stressful conditions. Diagnostic procedures units offer opportunities to link knowledge of anatomy with a patient's signs and symptoms and allow students to practice patient teaching and communication skills.

Although most nursing education programs eliminated an operating room clinical rotation from their curricula many years ago, learning to provide nursing care to patients who undergo surgery still is an important learning outcome. A scheduled or emergency surgical procedure is the reason for many hospital admissions, and because most nurses will encounter patients before or after their surgeries in home, community, or inpatient settings, students need to learn how to meet the needs of perioperative patients and their families. Students can learn aseptic technique effectively through such activities as performing a surgical scrub and establishing and maintaining a sterile field; once learned, these skills can be transferred to any other setting in which attention to sterile technique is important. The operating room also is an excellent setting for learning delegation, work organization, and teamwork skills. Follow-through activities that allow students to assess and teach a patient preoperatively, provide care in the circulator or scrub role intraoperatively, provide immediate postoperative care, and make a home visit to evaluate the patient's progress and outcomes of care are opportunities to understand continuity of health care.

Selecting acute care settings like these requires careful planning with nursing and other professional staff members. Students may need to be assigned individually instead of in groups, making the presence of an instructor with each student unlikely. Staff members might serve as preceptors for students, or specific guidelines for student involvement in patient care activities should be negotiated.

Ambulatory, Community, and Home Health Care Settings

Ambulatory, community, and home health care settings are potential sites for clinical learning activities when the learning objectives focus on wellness care, health promotion, patient and family teaching, monitoring of chronic health conditions, anticipatory guidance, and continuity of care. Ambulatory health learning activities can take place in public health and visiting nurse agencies, clinics, and physician, nurse practitioner, and nurse midwife practices. Home and community settings, including schools, day care centers, workplaces, camps, and retirement communities, are appropriate sites for emphasizing wellness care, health promotion, and population-based care. When learning objectives relate to health care for underserved populations, settings such as homeless and women's shelters, outreach centers, rural health centers, and soup kitchens might provide appropriate clinical activities.

Nurse-managed health centers often provide opportunities for students to practice primary health or wellness care. Nurse-managed centers may provide access to care for vulnerable populations as well as a focus on health promotion and disease prevention that allows students to explore and respond to a variety of needs. Hatcher, Scarinzi, and Kreider (1998) described the use of an urban nurse-managed health center as a clinical setting for undergraduate and graduate students in nursing, medicine, and social work. Students planned and implemented health promotion or disease prevention projects based on an assessment of a community population. Opportunities to collaborate with community organizations such as Head Start, schools, and soup kitchens exposed students to a primary health care model in action. Learning outcomes included the recognition that patients often must meet their nonmedical needs before they are able to follow recommended health care practices.

INNOVATIVE SELECTION AND USE OF CLINICAL SITES

Nursing faculty have reported numerous creative uses of traditional and nontraditional clinical settings. Selected examples of these innovations are described below.

LaSala and colleagues (1997) described the use of an interdisciplinary rural primary care center for clinical teaching of nursing, social work, health administration, health education, and premedicine students. The community was a rural county designated as a health professional shortage area. Learning activities occurred in the community hospital, home health care agency, public health department, primary medical care practice, community mental health center, and public schools. Students were invited to live in the community with practicing health professionals to increase their understanding of cultural factors that affected the health of the community.

Kavanagh (1998) portrayed the formation of a collaborative, caring community in a 6-week immersion learning experience for nursing students in High Plains Ogala Lakota tribal programs. Nursing students lived on the reservation and worked with tribal groups toward the groups' program goals, maximizing exposure to the tribal culture and minimizing contact with familiar bureaucratic organizations. These students collaborated with the faculty to develop a teaching/learning model that integrated diversity with caring in the context of developing cultural competence.

The use of summer camps for children with chronic conditions as clinical learning sites for students studying pediatric nursing was described by Praeger (1997). Strategies for identifying potential sites included seeking information from children's hospitals and nonprofit organizations whose mission was to serve children with special needs. Camps ranged from day camps for children with multiple handicaps who required total care to residential camps with a focus on recreation for children with a chronic illness. Selection of camps as clinical sites was based on a match between available learning opportunities and learning objectives that focused on use of the nursing process, decision making, growth and development, family dynamics, group process, ethical and legal aspects, and professional role relationships.

Another creative approach to choosing clinical sites for pediatric nursing practice was described by Hitt and Overbay (1997). A combination of sites was used to provide pediatric clinical learning activities based on a model of primary, secondary, and tertiary health promotion. The belief that comprehensive pediatric nursing is practiced in many places outside hospitals prompted a search for alternatives to the pediatric unit of the local community hospital. A combination of required and enrichment learning activities was planned. Required activities related to all three levels of health promotion; enrichment activities provided in-depth opportunities to meet individual learning needs and interests. Required primary health promotion activities took place in day care centers and preschools; enrichment activities were offered in a high school and at a health screening for home-schooled children. Required secondary health promotion activities in the community hospital pediatric unit allowed students to focus on care of the child with health deviations and the effect of the illness on the child and family; enrichment activities were offered at a burn unit, a pediatric intensive care unit, and an ambulatory surgery unit. The focus of tertiary health promotion activities was on the child with a chronic or terminal illness. Required learning activities were located in a pediatric rehabilitation hospital and a pediatric long-term-care facility; enrichment activities included extended opportunities in either of these facilities or making home visits to pediatric patients with a home health care nurse.

Arrington (1997) suggested that nursing education programs located in areas with large retirement communities have a rich source of potential clinical sites. A retirement community includes residents with a variety of lifestyles, physical abilities, and interests and therefore provides opportunities for nursing students to assess the commonalities and differences in an aging population. In this account of the use of a retirement community as a clinical site, nursing students participated in clinical learning activities under the guidance of a certified gerontological nurse in the position of health consultant who provided health promotion and health maintenance services. Learning objectives focused on developing communication and basic psychomotor skills; assessing mobility, safety concerns, vision and hearing deficits, and mental status; health education; and developing positive attitudes about the aging process.

Programs and facilities for homeless individuals and families provided clinical learning sites for graduate nursing students in an entry-level master's program described by Wolf, Goldfader, and Lehan (1997). Objectives included learning population-focused health promotion and communicating with people for whom trust and acceptance were challenging. Learning activities included performing a community assessment of an urban homeless community; assessing and providing care to homeless people in drop-in and day care programs, individual and family shelters, and a foot clinic for substance-abusing homeless men and women; and providing homeless women with opportunities for self-expression through a writing project. Students learned a broad definition of primary care and creative approaches to person-centered care.

Finally, advanced practice nurse faculty members related the use of two nurse-managed wellness centers as clinical learning sites (Resick, Taylor, Carroll, D'Antonio, & de Chesnay, 1997; Taylor, Resick, D'Antonio, & Carroll, 1997). Nurse-managed wellness clinics established in two urban elderly high-rise apartment buildings provided opportunities for faculty practice as well as clinical learning sites for undergraduate and graduate students in nursing, pharmacy, and occupational therapy. Learning activities varied according to the student's educational level and discipline and included health assessment, environmental assessment, health education, monitoring of chronic health problems, and support for self-care. These activities enabled students to meet learning objectives related to a wellness and health promotion model of care for elderly persons; promoting health, functioning, and quality of life for older adults; and developing positive attitudes toward elderly individuals. Graduate students preparing for roles as advanced practice nurses also benefited from the role modeling of the wellness center nurse managers.

SUMMARY

The goals of clinical learning may be accomplished in any environment where students can interact with patients: integrated health networks, homes, community centers, schools, workplaces, shelters, hospices, transitional and extended care facilities, day care centers, and the like. As the focus of health care becomes more global, wellness-oriented, and population-based, settings for the delivery of care become more diverse. Educating nursing students in such settings sensitizes them to the needs of diverse populations and enhances recruitment of nursing students to practice in underserved areas. This chapter discussed the transition to community care, interdisciplinary clinical education, and the increasing focus on global health care education. It also suggested innovative ways to use traditional and nontraditional settings to meet clinical learning objectives.

Patients increasingly are found outside acute care settings, in their homes and communities. Community-based activities help students to learn holistic care of individuals and families in the context of their communities and cultures and to identify community health needs and services and resources to meet them. "Community-based" may be interpreted in two ways: (1) a focus on the care of aggregate populations or community as client or (2) community-based nursing of patients with varying health problems. Patient care skills can be transferred from hospital to home settings to meet the needs of patients who were discharged after short inpatient stays. However, additional skills such as interpreting epidemiological data, building coalitions to address community problems, assessing community resources, and discerning the impact of environment on health are required for competent care of aggregate populations.

Successful transition to teaching and learning in community-based settings requires faculty and student preparation. Teachers who have little preparation in public health or community practice may require assistance in preparing to teach nursing care of aggregate populations. Teaching in this environment requires indirect guidance of student activities and a more collaborative teaching style that challenge long-held, implicit assumptions of how nurses must be prepared to practice. Before entering the community for clinical learning activities, students should practice patient teaching skills and solving ill-structured problems that are typical of those encountered in community settings. Student preparation also includes special attention to safety precautions.

The education of health care professionals is shifting from the traditional discipline-specific educational models to interdisciplinary education. The health care environment increasingly requires nurses to practice as members of multiprofessional teams, and student learning activities should resemble these practice realities. Interdisciplinary clinical education allows students of various health care professions to learn through shared experiences in the same settings, learning about the contributions of each discipline to patient care without competition. Clinical settings that are models of interdisciplinary practice, such as geriatric care centers, hospices, and rehabilitation centers, are excellent sites for clinical teaching in nursing.

Health problems extend beyond national borders, requiring a global view of health needs and health care. Nurses must develop sensitivity to cultural values, beliefs, and traditions in order to provide culturally appropriate care. Clinical learning sites in international health settings help students develop cultural sensitivity and competence as well as a global view of nursing and health care.

The selection of clinical learning activities should be based primarily on the learning objectives. Learning objectives can be achieved in a number of ways and should not prescribe a specific setting where the learning activities must take place. Creativity and flexibility in considering how objectives might be met will enable clinical teachers to identify a wide variety of clinical settings in which learning activities might occur. Learning activities can take place in acute care, ambulatory, community, and home health settings. Examples were given to illustrate the creative use of such clinical learning sites as operating rooms, nurse-managed wellness centers, rural primary care centers, and camps for children with chronic illnesses.

REFERENCES

Arrington, D. T. (1997). Retirement communities as creative clinical opportunities. *N & HC: Perspectives on Community, 18*, 82–85.

Bellack, J. P., Gerrity, P., Moore, S. M., Novotny, J., Quinn, D., Norman, L., & Harper, D. C. (1997). Taking aim at interdisciplinary education for continuous improvement in health care. *Nursing and Health Care Perspectives, 18*, 308–315.

Benson, J. A. (1997). Overcoming parochialism: Interdisciplinary training of the generalist team. *Nursing and Health Care Perspectives, 18*, 285.

Hatcher, P. A., Scarinzi, G. D., & Kreider, M. S. (1998). Meeting the need: A primary health care model for a community-based/nurse-managed health center. *Nursing and Health Care Perspectives, 19*, 12–19.

Henry, B. (1994). Nursing scholarship for world health. *Image: Journal of Nursing Scholarship, 26*, 170.

Hitt, S. F., & Overbay, J. D. (1997). Maximizing the possibilities: Pediatric nursing education in non-traditional settings. *Journal of Nursing Education, 36*, 339–341.

Hunt, R. (1998). Community-based nursing: Philosophy or setting? *American Journal of Nursing, 98*(10), 44–47.

Kavanagh, K. H. (1998). Summers of no return: Transforming care through a nursing field school. *Journal of Nursing Education, 37*, 71–79.

LaSala, K. B., Hopper, S. K., Rissmeyer, D. J., & Shipe, D. P. S. (1997). Rural health care and interdisciplinary education. *Nursing and Health Care Perspectives, 18*, 292–298.

Lockhart, J. S., & Resick, L. K. (1997). Teaching cultural competence: The value of experiential learning and community resources. *Nurse Educator, 22*(3), 27–31.

Mundt, M. H. (1997). A model for clinical learning experiences in integrated health care networks. *Journal of Nursing Education, 36*, 309–316.

Oneha, M. F., Magnussen, L., & Feletti, G. (1998). Ensuring quality nursing education in community-based settings. *Nurse Educator, 23*(1), 26–31.

Praeger, S. G. (1997). Establishing camps as clinical sites. *Journal of Nursing Education, 36*, 236–237.

Reed, F. C., & Wuyscik, M. A. (1998). Teach what?: Reflections on the transition from hospital teaching to teaching in the community. *Nurse Educator, 23*(1), 11–13.

Reilly, D. E., & Oermann, M. H. (1992). *Clinical teaching in nursing education* (2nd ed.). New York: National League for Nursing.

Resick, L. K., Taylor, C. A., Carroll, T. L., D'Antonio, J. A., & de Chesnay, M. (1997). Establishing a nurse-managed wellness clinic in a predominantly older African American inner-city high rise: An advanced practice nursing project. *Nursing Administration Quarterly, 21*(4), 47–54.

Ross, C. A. (1998). Preparing American and Nicaraguan nurses to practice home health nursing in a transcultural experience. *Home Health Care Management and Practice, 11*(1), 65–69.

Ryan, S. A., D'Aoust, R. F., Groth, S., McGee, K., & Small, A. L. (1997). A faculty on the move into the community. *Nursing and Health Care Perspectives, 18*, 139–141, 149.

Stokes, L. (1998). Teaching in the clinical setting. In D. M. Billings & J. A. Halstead (Eds.), *Teaching in nursing: A guide for faculty* (pp. 281–297). Philadelphia: Saunders.

Taylor, C. A., Resick, L., D'Antonio, J. A., & Carroll, T. L. (1997). The advanced practice nurse role in implementing and evaluating two nurse-managed wellness clinics: Lessons learned about structure, process, and outcomes. *Advanced Practice Nursing Quarterly, 3*(2), 36–45.

Virgin, S. E., & Goodrow, B. (1997). A community crossword puzzle: An interdisciplinary approach to community-based learning. *Nursing and Health Care Perspectives, 18,* 302–307.

Wolf, K. A., Goldfader, R., & Lehan, C. (1997). Women speak: Healing the wounds of homelessness through writing. *N & HC: Perspectives on Community, 18,* 74–78.

Index

Springer Publishing Company

Interactive Group Learning
Strategies for Nurse Educators
Deborah L. Ulrich, PhD, RN,
Kellie J. Glendon, MSN, RN, C

Two experienced nurse educators have created a handbook of strategies that instructors can implement now to create a dynamic group learning environment for today's student nurses. Every chapter shows how to implement innovative, cooperative group learning: the emphasis is on teaching applications that yield both critical thinking and comprehension in students. These are workshop tested techniques that stand on a foundation of group learning theory. The authors show how to combine writing exercises, cooperative learning, reviews, and new testing formats into their Comprehensive Group Learning Model.

To assist nursing educators and students, this handbook contains over 55 useful illustrations that help demonstrate new ideas for teaching and interactive group learning.

Contents: Introduction • Changing Classroom Dynamics for theNew Learning Paradigm • An Experiential Comprehensive Group Learning Model • Using Cooperative Learning Strategies in Nursing • Strategies to Connect Students Holistically • Group Structures for Preparation and Review • Writing As a Tool for Critical Thinking • Putting It All Together and Implementing Group Learning Strategies: Issues for Faculty and Students • References

1999   136pp.   0-8261-1238-2   hardcover

536 Broadway, New York, NY 10012-3955 • (212) 431-4370 • Fax (212) 941-7842